The Health Revolution

Give Yourself the Healthcare You Deserve

PRAISE FOR DR. JADE WIMBERLEY

"Dr. Jade is a true lifesaver. Yes, in a 'Toss me a flotation device, I'm drowning!' kind of way, but also in a 'Let's build a boat to cross this wide ocean safely together' way. She has come to my rescue during acute health crises when the waters got too high and shored up my leaky vessel to make it more seaworthy generally. This is a rare and potent combination—a provider who is good in moments of acute need and in developing preventative measures. I've dealt with challenging mental health issues for most of my adult life, balancing a high-powered career and high-octane ambition with difficult neurobiology. Dr. Jade has both provided me with helpful nutritional recommendations and other care guidance directly, as well as pivotal connections to other practitioners within her network. She is a brilliant integrative doctor and a beautiful soul; my life—and health—are better for having known and worked with her. I'd let her captain my ship anytime."

—**K.D.**, Environmental Policy Director and Activist, Oakland, CA

"At the age of 59, I sought out Dr. Jade Wimberley's consultation to help monitor my aging process by interpreting blood tests and boosting my system with vitamin-mineral drips. She is pragmatic, and asked me interesting questions like: 'How are you sleeping?' and 'How are you pooping?' She is present. Her bedside manner is assuring. Dr. Wimberley is keenly interested in the complexities of the human organism and tends to not rush to a conclusion. She is an advocate of the ancient medical models in which one went to the doctor to maintain one's health, as opposed to putting it off until the dis-ease was fully developed. Through our consultations, I developed a deeper trust and knowing of my body's ability to heal itself."

—**Matthew Engelhart**, co-owner of Cafe Gratitude and Gracias Madre restaurants, author, free-thinker, husband, father, and grandfather.

"Dr. Wimberley walks what she talks and lives what she believes. This is a true case where her life imitates her art and we all benefit from it."

– **Dr. Holly Lucille**, ND,RN, Los Angeles, CA

"In May 2014, I was diagnosed with Anaplastic Carcinoma Thyroid Cancer, which is an extremely rare cancer, known to be aggressive and resistant to treatment. My family suggested I work with Dr. Jade Wimberley for a regimen of many nutritional infusions to support my immune system and overall health while I underwent chemotherapy and radiation treatments. [Dr. Wimberley] encouraged me to believe in the healing power of the body and mind through such a trying time. I am now 18 months out from diagnosis and so far cancer free. This experience left me believing in the need for more integrative healthcare especially with advanced disease states. She certainly helped me achieve good health again in my life."

—**J.G.**, Berkeley, CA

The Health Revolution

Give Yourself the Healthcare You Deserve

Dr. Jade Wimberley

LUX
BOOKS

Published and distributed by:
Lux Books
1372 West Main Street
Carbondale, Colorado 81623
(970) 510-5394
office@luxwellnesscenter.com
LuxWellnessCenter.com

Contact us for author interviews or speaking engagements.

First Edition

ISBN: 9780692928028

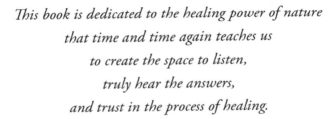

This book is dedicated to the healing power of nature
that time and time again teaches us
to create the space to listen,
truly hear the answers,
and trust in the process of healing.

Table of Contents

Foreword

When I first met Dr. Jade, I found her warm, friendly, and professional manner very appealing. As I overheard her speaking to other guests at one of our farm dinners, I kept thinking what a kind and interested woman she is. I also remember thinking, when I learned she was a doctor, WOW! what a great combination—a doctor who takes time to truly listen and who really cares.

Having become a patient of hers, I can now say that is exactly who she is: a caring, attentive, and empowering healer. She is always thoughtful, letting you be in control of your own health, and yet informing you regarding the choices you have. I am amazed at Dr. Jade's ability to gently guide my attention toward my health goals. Life is busy, and I find myself not always putting my health in its rightful place in the pecking order.

I turned to Dr. Jade when my primary physician was unwilling to continue prescribing the hormones I'd been taking. We had been experimenting with the available strength and found nothing that would work for me. Dr. Jade, on the other hand, requested additional blood work. She evaluated the lab results and advised me about supplements and alternative bioidentical hormones that would work. She was able to dial in to exactly what my body needed and wanted. Her prescription quickly impacted my energy level and confidence in my well-being. She peacefully moved my emotions from confusion and frustration to clarity and excitement.

I was a fairly healthy woman in my sixties when we first met, and now I am a very healthy woman closer to seventy. I have never felt so empowered in my own body as I do now.

When Dr. Jade asked me to read this book and write the foreword, I immediately and selfishly said, "Yes," because I wanted to be on the cutting edge of her cutting edge!

What I love about this book is how easy it is to apply the wisdom. It makes proactive well-being as an alternative to managing illness readily available and simplifies the task of sifting through medical jargon. I've heard too many frustrating stories regarding healthcare, and know how powerless I felt as I searched for means to continue my own good health. I've come to understand that if we all learn to take more responsibility for the way our health is handled and apply the guidelines in this book, we will heal ourselves. As more of us experience this healing, the Earth will become healthy again, too. This is why The Health Revolution is a worthy personal and social cause to take up.

This book is wonderful. I mean that. It is full of wonder in the form of insight, knowledge, options, clarity, empowerment, and sound advice to lead you on your healing health journey.

Terces Engelhart
Author, blogger, restaurateur, business consultant, and lifestyle coach

Introduction

The art, music, and cultural movements of the 1960s in America are at the very least iconic. The social protests regarding sex, race, war, and a variety of freedoms in that decade changed us and the world we inhabit. The time we live in today, let's call it the time around 2020, will birth yet another significant Cultural Revolution—The Health Revolution.

People feel trapped by our existing healthcare system and are crying out, once again, for freedom. They want to be free to choose their healthcare providers, including alternative healthcare. They want that care to be affordable and accessible, and they want to be their own best-informed healthcare advocate. The unrest in our country over the way we approach health and healthcare, is justifiably snowballing. It is time to do something about it.

I remember vividly a conversation with my grandmother on her back porch in the summer of 1998. It was a typical humid Baltimore morning with the birds chirping as if they wanted us to serve them breakfast, too. We were eating my grandmother's infamous thinly sliced toast, topped with marmalade purchased from the farmers market, and enjoying a cup of coffee while catching up with one another. At the time, I lived on Bainbridge Island, Washington, so we only saw one another two or three times a year. That was the day I told my grandmother, whom I revered, that I was going to naturopathic medical school. Taken aback she said, "Jade, why don't you go to real medical school and make it easier on yourself?" Although those words were a stab in my heart, they did not penetrate deeply enough to deter me. I had chosen a path less traveled by most healthcare practitioners, but then and now, I have no doubt that the medicine of the future will be based on health and wellness and not disease management.

My decision to go to naturopathic medical school had come after an anaphylactic reaction to allergy shots that I had been receiving regularly for 12 years. The allergy symptoms and subsequent reaction to the treatment were physically daunting, but they also drained me emotionally and spiritually. I was at a physical and spiritual tipping point, and that's when I had my first aha moment. I realized the healthcare status quo was not working for me. It was time for a radical change in the way I was approaching my health. I felt there had to be other options for obtaining balanced health, and with it a better quality of life. For that reason, I embarked on a career path that led me to become a naturopathic doctor.

My journey toward living a fulfilling, health-filled life began those many years ago, but is not yet complete. There is so much more change needed regarding our healthcare, and that's why I have initiated The Health Revolution. Every day, I hear from patients who seem fed up with the lack of true concern from their doctors and the knee-jerk prescribing of medications. They tell me stories of doctors rolling their eyes when the patient asks if nutrition plays a role in their conditions, or if there is something other than medications they can use effectively. Masking symptoms with medications may have satisfied patients for decades, but today, patients are demanding integrated care and are less enamored with managing disease; they want to prevent disease. What's more, they desire to feel their very best at all stages of life. The tide is changing, and as a result, the days of ten-minute appointments, over-prescribing of medications, and lack of nutritional and preventative education will soon be obsolete.

I have the privilege and obligation as a naturopathic doctor to spend time with patients and educate them about the roles lifestyle and nutrition play in maintaining health. I discuss alternatives to medications when applicable. I suggest books to read, podcasts to enjoy, and actions to take such as relaxation, diet, exercise, and education that can ignite personal Health Revolutions. I do this because it is what I pledged to do as a doctor. But even more fulfilling for me, I do it because I love nudging, guiding, and witnessing patients as they become more informed and wake up to all the possibilities of their potential.

My practice, website, and this book are my ways of empowering all my patients, and you, so that you can get ahead of disease, make beneficial health choices, and do more easily what matters to you.

You will find within these pages eight health-restoring tenets. These are the actions that benefit my patients most in their quest to live longer, more fulfilled lives replete with love, community, nature, and delicious food. This book is meant to raise awareness and provide readers with a basic foundation on which to build their very own health-care team and practice. It is an introduction to alternative healthcare choices only and not a definitive diet book or methodology. I have endeavored to provide additional resources and to cite sources for much of the information I have provided. Ultimately, I wish simply to relay what has been successful in my practice—the information and efforts that have helped my patients thrive.

And so, I welcome you to become part of The Health Revolution, so that we can all work together to change the way we do health in America.

Sincerely,

Jade Wimberley, ND

Dr. Jade Wimberley

CHAPTER 1

The Revolution Revelation

If I had superpowers, I would *ZAP!* the way we do health in America. As a mere mortal with a medical degree, however, the extent of my magic is to provide education that will restore what is innately your right—a system in which wellness care is prioritized over disease management. This book has the purpose of helping you give yourself the healthcare you deserve.

I see it weekly in my practice. New patients come to me tired, sick, and emotionally downtrodden. They have tried unsuccessfully to find wellness and a bit of comfort within the existing healthcare system. The stories they impart regarding the lack of effective and concerned care they have received from health practitioners prior to crossing my threshold saddens and angers me. As I see it, the Western medical paradigm is less than perfect. Amidst the Food and Drug Administration (FDA), insurance companies, hospitals, pharmaceutical companies, pharmacies, and the American Medical Association (AMA), a system has developed that serves not the patient and their wellness, but the system itself and greedy individuals who exploit it.

Our current Western medical framework follows the "business-as-usual" approach. "It has always been done that way and it will stay that way," seems to be the general attitude. This modus operandi will not change unless we do something about it. It's time to shed light on how ineffective and harmful the status quo has become. It's time for The Health Revolution.

GOALS OF THE HEALTH REVOLUTION

We are on the brink of a consciousness shift in America regarding the state of our healthcare. As our country faces epidemics of obesity, cancer, and diabetes; as we become more resistant to antibiotics; as we realize that we are too often stressed and tired, it appears that mainstream medicine continues to ignore our request for a new system. I am not just talking about the political debate as to whether or not we should have socialized medicine; I'm talking about a fundamental, grassroots movement that will redesign the type of care offered to patients today.

Why, for example, does mainstream medicine refuse to offer nutrition as a viable way to heal? Why do doctors who treat diabetes continue to have jellybeans, chocolate, and donuts in their offices when these are the things that perpetuate the disease? Why do doctors spend ten minutes or

GOALS OF THE HEALTH REVOLUTION

- Create community and a forum for discussion providing an avenue to change.

- Challenge the existing "fix the disease" medical model.

- Develop preventative and holistic healthcare alternatives that are readily available and affordable.

- Educate people about how they can truly be healthy.

- Empower people to take control of their own health.

- Establish availability of affordable, nutrient-dense, organic food grown by community farmers.

- Heal the Earth so the Earth can continue to nurture and heal us.

less talking to us and ignore lifestyle and stress factors before prescribing a pill? We, the people, should be demanding healthcare options other than medication, surgery, and more medication. We deserve to be heard and receive an affordable, safe, and effective response from our doctors and our politicians.

Since the Affordable Care Act of 2010, the states of Alaska, Hawaii, Oregon, Vermont, and Washington have taken the lead in this quest. They've teamed up with insurance companies that include licensed naturopathic doctors in their networks, providing consumers more choice. Insurance companies that have been compliant are Premera Blue Cross, Regence, First Choice Health, Aetna, Cigna, Uniform, United, and Group Health. If we are going to be strong-armed into insurance policies, then we must be allowed to choose the type of provider with whom we are comfortable, including functional medicine doctors, chiropractors, acupuncturists, naturopathic doctors, and other alternative healthcare professionals.

It's time to talk out loud and demand real change in the types of healthcare available and ways we receive these services in the United States—hence, a revolution.

CHALLENGE THE STATUS QUO

Most of us have been raised on the Western medical model and going to the doctor with a follow up visit to the pharmacy for our medicine is just what we do. We often continue this cycle without ever discovering and treating the root source of the ailment. I encounter new patients regularly who are taking numerous medications and whose overall health is mismanaged by two or three doctors who rarely have the time to get to know their patients.

In the past 15 years, prescription rates for antipsychotics in children have increased fivefold.[1] In my practice, I am seeing a marked increase in the number of teen patients who have been prescribed antipsychotics to aid their sleep, prior to turning to me. Prescribing an antipsychotic to a teen as a sleep aid should be a criminal offense! Apparently, it's easier to hand out a prescription than to have a dialogue with the patient and understand why he is unable to sleep. If more time could be dedicated to talking it through with the patient and digging a little deeper, then perhaps a natural, healthful substitute could be offered. But there are several roadblocks to this type of care, and one of them is money. Oftentimes, insurance companies do not reimburse for in-depth doctor/patient dialogue, but they do reimburse for a diagnosis that is followed by medication.

A year and a half ago, a friend was diagnosed with stage-four colon and liver cancer with possible ovarian metastases. She was told by her first oncologist to put her life in order and given less than three months to live. Just like that, cut and dried.

The oncologist offered one option and that was to begin chemotherapy immediately, which he said would most likely do no good. He provided my friend with no incentive to fight for her life. But she had the insight to seek a more integrative approach and fight for a longer life. She put together a team of healthcare practitioners that reinforced

---

1. Gardiner Harris, "Use of Antipsychotics in Children Is Criticized," *The New York Times*, November 18, 2008, accessed November 19, 2008, http://www.nytimes.com/2008/11/19/health/policy/19fda.html.

her right to live. The team consisted of a more progressive medical oncologist, a naturopathic oncologist, radiologist, surgeon, psychologist, chiropractor, a personal trainer, close family, and a loving partner. Her team worked collectively and created a plan that highlighted the option to live even if it was going to be for a limited amount of time. With great remorse, I must share that 19 months after her initial diagnosis my dear friend passed away from cancer. Though she was too young (age 53) and not ready to leave her loved ones, she passed with dignity and felt she had done everything she could to prolong her life. She lived fully and with purpose for 19 months. She didn't die without hope in three. Many doctors would do well to pay more attention to how the news of terminal illness and the manner of their delivery of this news affects their patients. More common than not, when one is navigating cancer, medication and chemotherapy agents may play a role, but so do the medicine arts of Hippocrates' day[2], particularly "treading with care in matters of life and death" and employing preventative medicine. Too often, the latter two are overlooked and the former given as the only option to wellness.

I am saddened by the impersonal, ineffective care my friend received and by how low the standard of Western medical practice has become. It makes me even sadder that

---

2. Hippocrates, a Greek physician born circa 460 BCE, is considered by many as the father of medicine and medical ethical standards. About 60 medical writings bear his name, including the Hippocratic Oath. However, contemporary scholars question whether or not Hippocrates truly was the author. Compiled from https://www.britannica.com/biography/Hippocrates.

HIPPOCRATIC OATH, MODERN VERSION

I swear to fulfill, to the best of my ability and judgment, this covenant: • I will respect the hard-won scientific gains of those physicians in whose steps I walk, and gladly share such knowledge as is mine with those who are to follow. • I will apply, for the benefit of the sick, all measures which are required, avoiding those twin traps of overtreatment and therapeutic nihilism. • I will remember that there is art to medicine as well as science, and that warmth, sympathy, and understanding may outweigh the surgeon's knife or the chemist's drug. • I will not be ashamed to say "I know not," nor will I fail to call in my colleagues when the skills of another are needed for a patient's recovery. • I will respect the privacy of my patients, for their problems are not disclosed to me that the world may know. Most especially must I tread with care in matters of life and death. If it is given me to save a life, all thanks. But it may also be within my power to take a life; this awesome responsibility must be faced with great humbleness and awareness of my own frailty. Above all, I must not play at God. • I will remember that I do not treat a fever chart, a cancerous growth, but a sick human being, whose illness may affect the person's family and economic stability. My responsibility includes these related problems, if I am to care adequately for the sick. • I will prevent disease whenever I can, for prevention is preferable to cure. • I will remember that I remain a member of society, with special obligations to all my fellow human beings, those sound of mind and body as well as the infirm. • If I do not violate this oath, may I enjoy life and art, respected while I live and remembered with affection thereafter. May I always act so as to preserve the finest traditions of my calling and may I long experience the joy of healing those who seek my help. • *Written in 1964 by Louis Lasagna, Academic Dean of the School of Medicine at Tufts University, and used in many medical schools today.*

we are doing so little about it. We often receive misguided care from the current "business as usual" medical model because we are not ready as a society to confront this seemingly overwhelming healthcare issue. This has to change. We cannot continue to wait for the system to change of its own volition. We need to effect the change by demanding and participating in the following:

- Patronize healthcare practitioners who spend enough time with patients to educate and treat the whole person, not just the disease.

- Insist that patients be allowed to choose their doctors. Americans are now required to have health insurance, so let's insist on the right to choose the type of practitioner with whom we partner.

- Eliminate the incentive for doctors to over-test patients primarily because they are reimbursed by insurance companies.

- Require at least two expert opinions before allowing non-urgent surgical procedures. Too many unnecessary procedures and surgeries increase healthcare costs.

- Recognize that over-processed food may be the root of our illnesses and that real food is medicine. Real food has the ability to often CURE chronic diseases such as diabetes, obesity, and asthma. Many disease states are curable.

- Separate pharmaceutical companies and medical school funding.

- Separate the Food Administration from the Drug Administration.

- Prohibit pharmaceutical ads on TV.

The Nielsen Company has determined that there are, on average, 80 drug commercials every hour of every day represented on television.[3] When 80 drug commercials an hour have the potential to bombard us, it is nearly impossible not to believe that drugs will cure all our health maladies. Drugs can be, at times, part of the healthcare picture but by no means are they the only pathway to health. Let's replace drug-endorsing commercials with public service announcements that encourage a health-conscious lifestyle, including real food diets, stress management, exercise, and a supportive community.

At present, we do not have an effective preventative healthcare system in the United States. We have a reactive, disease care system. We offer quick fixes in the form of pills, syrups, and creams. It's always the same answer: "Take this for that." By the time someone is 40 years old, he's on four medications, by his fiftieth birthday, it's five meds, and by age 60, six meds. This is a habit The Health Revolution can help conscientious patients and healthcare practitioners break.

3. Alix Spiegel, "Selling Sickness: How Drug Ads Changed Health Care," NPR Special Series, updated October 13, 2009, accessed January 21, 2016, http://www.npr.org/templates/story/story.php?storyId=113675737.

SHIFT TO PREVENTATIVE CARE

The solution to this healthcare crisis is to shift the paradigm from our current sick and reactive healthcare model to a preventative one. We need to break down the existing medical model, keep what is good (such as surgery to reattach a finger that has been cut off), and then add what is missing: food as medicine, treating the whole person, availability, affordability, and a true desire to help. We need to make an investment in humanity, and not make money off the sick. Let's put more resources into preventing depression and anxiety, heart disease, high cholesterol, diabetes, obesity, hypothyroidism, and cancer. By resources, I mean money, compassionate doctors, and educators who actually reinforce dialogue and offer real food as part of the solution. Let's look at new approaches to medical research besides the antiquated, double-blind placebo controlled studies that are mostly funded by pharmaceutical giants with special interests. Let's break the habit of reaching for the prescription pad for everything from sleeplessness to low libido, and start writing RXs for fitness and nutrition classes, connection with nature, filtered drinking water, a naturally induced night's sleep, and creating supportive communities.

Truly, what are we waiting for? Let's start the ball rolling with conversation and raise more awareness. Together, let's build a system that fosters preventative health, education, and the power of choice.

FOOD FOR THOUGHT

I have a patient who, while suffering from gastrointestinal distress and severe pain in the hospital, was fed a liquid "food" containing high-fructose corn syrup, preservatives, and many other ingredients few of us can pronounce. This is standard practice because corporations making such "food" products contract with hospitals and insurance companies allowing for few, if any, alternatives. It's appalling that in many cases organic whole food is available to the hospital and ultimately the patient, but insurance companies will not reimburse for such options. This is hard to "digest" because it is known that corn syrup will only perpetuate the disease state, especially a gastrointestinal issue of unknown cause.

Processed foods and soft drinks are loaded with high-fructose corn syrup, and the enormous consumption of this type of food in the American diet has paralleled the rise in obesity and is associated with nonalcoholic fatty liver disease.[4] So why do hospitals (centers for healing) across the country still feed this sludge to sick patients? This is the type of question we should all be asking insistently.

Real food is the most profound medicine—it helps prevent illness and it heals. Disease diminishes and health is regained when we eat a diet that helps the bodily systems

4. George A. Bray, MD, "Potential Health Risks From Beverages Containing Fructose Found in Sugar or High-Fructose Corn Syrup," Diabetes Journals, accessed January 22, 2016, http://care.diabetesjournals. org/content/36/1/11.full.

stay in balance. This means a diet consisting of more vegetables, proteins, and healthy fats, instead of empty carbohydrates, processed foods, and high-fructose corn syrup. A person can make huge strides in improving her health by taking baby steps in changing her diet. For starters, one can substitute those two or three daily sodas or caffeine-laden energy drinks with

REAL FOOD IS THE MOST PROFOUND MEDICINE.

water. If this proves difficult, begin with homemade iced tea lightly sweetened, then unsweetened, then switch to herbal tea, and then plain old delicious water.

Some foods, such as processed, store-bought junk (donuts, corn puffs, hot dogs), we know are unhealthy choices for everyone. They don't truly feed our cells—they deplete them. But each of us is unique and our bodies may or may not work well with certain types of real food as well.

I discuss diet with every patient who steps across my threshold. I want to know what they drink and eat every day to see if there might be a dietary connection to what ails them. Many of us are unaware of what we consume and often surprised when we do stop and take notice. A food diary or related app offers perspective and insight with which to make changes. When you see what you've consumed in black and white, it's easier to connect the dots between symptoms and the food that is the source of your discomfort. You may realize that your migraine headaches come after consuming diet soda and a protein bar for lunch, or that you bloat and fart after eating corn tortillas or popcorn. Perhaps nightshade fruits and vegetables such as tomatoes, potatoes, peppers, and eggplant are causing the irritating rash on your forearm and stomach. Diet awareness and consumption of real food is an undeniable cornerstone for building health.

DEFINING ORGANIC AND GMO

"We are what we eat," Hippocrates said, and as I say, "We are what our food eats as well." Ideally, everyone would consume an organic diet. When we eat organic fruits, veggies, and sustainable animal products, we stay healthier. We eat nutrients, not toxins. A recent study published in the *British Journal of Nutrition* revealed that organic meat and milk contain 50 percent more omega-3 fatty acids and lower concentrations of saturated fats than conventional products, due mostly to the fact that organically raised animals eat grass and not cereal.[5]

Many patients often report that they eat less food once they switch to a more whole food-based diet versus the "Standard American Diet" (SAD). Patients eating real organic food consume calories that are nutrient-dense, and this stops cravings. Our body is happy, not sad. It's fulfilled.

5. "Organic Meat and Milk Contain 50% More Omega-3, Study Finds," Irish Examiner, February 16, 2016, accessed February 21, 2016, http://www.irishexaminer.com/examviral/science-world/organic-meat-and-milk-contain-50-more-omega-3-study-finds-382264.html.

Very specific criteria are in place for a food to be labeled USDA certified organic. In general, to qualify, a food must be grown and processed according to federal guidelines that address soil quality, fertilizers, pest and weed control, how animals are raised, and more. Visit the USDA website and/or blogs for more in-depth information.[6]

USDA certified organic food cannot be a genetically modified organism (GMO). Therefore, if you eat anything organic, it is not a GMO. However, a food can be labeled as non-GMO and not be organic. Confusing, right? And sometimes extremely misleading.

GMO crops such as soy, corn, and wheat make up the bulk of all processed foods in America, and federal law states that food manufacturers do not need to label this. These genetically modified foods allow chemical companies, agribusiness, and processed food giants to sell nutritionally empty, caloric products, and, consequently, perpetuate a vicious cycle of illness. While scientists, politicians, corporations, and consumers debate whether GMOs are safe for human consumption, we remain the uninformed lab rats. Let's remember that at one point in history we were all told that DDT and PCBs were "safe." Non-organic food is typically GMO, often consisting of added hormones, antibiotics, and preservatives. Simply put, it is not nourishing, but harmful to the body.

6. Miles McEvoy, National Organic Program Deputy Administrator, March 22, 2013 (11:00 a.m.), "Organic 101: What the USDA Organic Label Means," http://blogs.usda.gov/2012/03/22/organic-101-what-the-usda-organic-label-means/.

THE ECONOMIC FACTOR

Before I go further, I would like to discuss the belief that buying organic is too expensive, especially for the average family. While a non-GMO apple at the farmers market may cost more than one bought on sale at a chain grocery store, at the farmers market you will be less able to buy cookies, potato chips, canned sauces, and prepared frozen foods. You are less seduced by processed foods that do nothing but rob you of health. I don't discount that organic food comes with a higher price tag or that budgets are a significant consideration, but I do encourage you to look at possible long-term costs of being sick. Invest in good food now, and you will be far less likely to have medical bills, obese children, lost time at work, and rotten days where you feel like something the cat dragged in.

It's also worth noting the positive economic ripple effect in your community when you choose to shop at the local farmers market, instead of a large chain store. Research conducted by The Farmers Market Coalition reveals that monies spent at a farmers market are more likely to stay in the local economy versus monies spent at a large grocery chain. They state that, "for every 100 dollars spent at a farmers market, 62 dollars stay in the local economy and 99 dollars in the state."[7] Every day, we have the freedom to choose where we spend our food dollars. If we demand that

7. Farmers Market Coalition, "Farmers Markets Stimulate Local Economies," accessed July 10, 2016, https://farmersmarketcoalition.org/education/stimulate-local-economies-2/.

it be local and organic, companies will work with farmers and supply it. As organic and local becomes the food of choice, it will also become more affordable. A 2007 Harris poll indicated that 30 percent of Americans buy organic food at least on occasion, and believe that it is healthier, safer to eat, and better for the environment.[8]

As Hippocrates said, "Food is our medicine." I don't think he would have considered chemicals, pesticides, herbicides, fungicides, hormones, antibiotics, high-fructose corn syrup, and hydrogenated oils medicine. There is nothing therapeutic in overly processed food. The gut is especially susceptible to the potential dangers of GMO food. Bt (Bacillus thuringiensis) toxin, a pesticide produced by some genetically modified crops, has been shown with GMO corn consumption to significantly alter immune function in mice, and may cause disrupted immune function in the gut.[9] Monsanto, a leading and controversial GMO seed producer, has conducted research, as has an independent lab in France that determined that mice and rats eating Bt toxin-producing corn sustained liver and kidney damage.[10]

8. Mark Bittman, "Eating Food That's Better for You, Organic or Not," The New York Times, March 21, 2009, accessed March 26, 2009, http://www.nytimes.com/2009/03/22/weekinreview/22bittman.html.

9. R.I. Vázquez, L. Moreno-Fierros, L. Neri-Bazán, G.A. De La Riva, and R. López-Revilla,"Bacillus Thuringiensis Cry1Ac Protoxin Is a Potent Systemic and Mucosal Adjuvant," (Center for Genetic Engineering and Biotechnology, Havana, Cuba), PubMed.gov, June 1999, accessed May 11, 2016, http://www.ncbi.nlm.nih.gov/pubmed/10354369.

10. Joël Spiroux de Vendômois, François Roullier, Dominique Cellier, and Gilles-Eric Séralini, "A Comparison of the Effects of Three GM Corn

An integral component of The Health Revolution is making what you eat a top priority. It may be a giant leap for you to stop the weekly supermarket run and find a farmers market, but perhaps you can begin with baby steps. Buy organic whenever possible. If you learn of a local farmers market or summertime farm stand, take a field trip. Give up fat-free cookies and diet soda. With each step you take, you will reward yourself with better health.

FEEDING A PLANET

Genetic mutation will not be the solution to feeding an over-populated world. GMO agribusiness can only lead to more rapid destruction of our already fragile planet. Planting GMO mono-crops across vast lands rob the soil of nutrients and offer little nutritional value in return. Such "farming" is all about volume, sales of seeds, and the pesticides and herbicides that go with them.

A 2013 United Nations Farming Report says fairly clearly that organic and small-scale farming is the answer when it comes to feeding the world, not GMOs and

Varieties on Mammalian Health," International Journal of Biological Sciences 2009, accessed May 11, 2016, http://www.ijbs.com/v05p0706.htm.

Gilles-Eric Séralini, Dominique Cellier, and Joël Spiroux de Vendomois, "New Analysis of a Rat Feeding Study with a Genetically Modified Maize Reveals Signs of Hepatorenal Toxicity," Archives of Environmental Contamination and Toxicology, March 13, 2007, accessed May 11, 2016, http://ww.w.rapaluruguay.org/transgenicos/Maiz/Genetically_Maize.pdf.

monoculture.[11] We can expedite this solution if we economically support farmers who are using non-GMO seeds and farming practices. It would be beneficial for humans, animals, ecosystems—the entire planet—for our food supply to be based on local farming and local distribution. The more we purchase non-GMO (and organic if possible), the more grass roots farmers (not corporations) will grow it. Over the past ten years, farmers markets have grown exponentially. The USDA reports there are 8,144 markets now listed in the National Farmers Market Directory.[12] That's up from 5,000 in 2008, and that's welcome news!

Communities growing their own organic food are one long-term solution to the lack of nutritious food, starvation, and the restoration of our planet. I'm talking about regional agriculture grown in fertile (not depleted) soil within a 50-mile radius of where one lives. Let's provide tax incentives for communities to grow their own food. Let's assist local farmers to grow, not only in rural areas but also in urban environments, on the sides of buildings, rooftops, and on reclaimed and cleaned up abandoned lots. Or, for pleasure, exercise, and a natural dose of sunshiny vitamin D, grow food in your very own garden.

---

11. "Wake up Before It's Too Late," Trade and Environment Review 2013: UN Commission on Trade and Environment publication, accessed December 9, 2015, http://unctad.org/en/PublicationsLibrary/ditcted2012d3_en.pdf.

12. "USDA Celebrates National Farmers Market Week, August 4-10," accessed April 15, 2015, http://www.usda.gov/wps/portal/usda/usdahome?contentid=2013/08/0155.xml.

It boils down to this: real food is medicine and GMO processed gunk perpetuates disease. Diverse, local agriculture nourishes and heals the Earth and us. Agribusiness and GMO pollute. To me this is an easy choice to make and a valid reason to incite this revolution.

CHANGE ISN'T COMFORTABLE

The issue, of course, lies in the fact that change is often uncomfortable. Do you want to change your eating and living patterns, or do you just want to take a pill? Do you want to make a trip to the farmers market on the weekend and cook, or do you want to stop at the drive-through window and gobble a greasy burger while driving home after a long workday? To change the status quo, we may need to accept being a little bit uncomfortable.

CHAPTER 1 HEALTH RESOLUTION

What can you change in your life that will affect your health and the greater community? Reading this book is a great first step. You may also want to reflect on how the current healthcare system does or doesn't serve you.

1. Jot down a list of what isn't working for you regarding the status quo of healthcare. Perhaps it's the fact that your insurance company won't pay for a consultation with a nutritionist or that your doctor makes you wait an hour in the office, and your examination and diagnosis takes ten minutes. Perhaps you want to know more about why you feel so exhausted all the time. Maybe you want your local grade school to remove the soda machine from the cafeteria.

2. Take a moment and resolve to take one small action regarding one of the issues on your list. For example: I, for both personal reasons and because I am a naturopathic doctor, want GMO foods to be clearly labeled. I am going to educate my patients on the importance of this health-related and political issue.

Lots of tiny steps can take The Health Revolution a long distance. Every voice added to the choir will create a song that has to be heard.

CHAPTER 2

Doctoring and the Health Revolution

Revolutions often have an underlying theme of empower-ment. As a naturopathic doctor, patient education is ex-tremely important to me. I can serve patients best when they understand what is happening in their bodies because they can then become their own best health advocates. This chapter is all about empowerment and steps patients can take to find true preventative care that includes high regard for the individual.

Because there is so much interest in a new system of medical treatment, there are many terms bandied about when it comes to alternative healthcare. To clarify these terms and empower you as you make healthcare choices, here are some helpful definitions:

HEALTHCARE PRACTITIONER, ABBREVIATION, & DEFINITION

Acupuncture (LAc) is a system of medicine originating in ancient China that alleviates pain and treats physical and emotional health issues by inserting fine needles into the body's "energy highways" known as meridians.

Allopathic Medicine (MD) is a term used by alternative medicine practitioners referring to mainstream medicine that treats or suppresses disease by the use of drugs or surgery.

Alternative Medicine offers a variety of treatments that are an "alternative" to the Western medical approach (hospitals, medications, surgeries). It is more of a vague marketing term, and has little meaning to any particular type of practice.

Ayurvedic Medicine originated in India over 3,000 years ago and accordingly is one of the world's oldest medical systems. It is a holistic approach based on the idea that good health is achieved when body, mind, and spirit are in harmony and connected to the universe. Treatments include but are not limited to herbs, diet, massage, breathwork, meditation, and yoga.

Traditional Chinese/Oriental Medicine is an ancient medicinal system from China employing acupuncture, Chinese herbs, massage, dietary therapy, and martial arts as part of the healing process. A basic premise is that the body's *chi*, or vital energy, circulates through meridians that branch out and have connections to the organs and to their functions.

Chiropractic Medicine (DC) frees the spinal column of subluxations, allowing the muscular and nervous systems to move more freely.

Complementary Medicine is an alternative treatment form that works in conjunction with traditional medicine. For example, a cancer patient may have an oncologist and an acupuncturist to help with the side effects of chemotherapy. The acupuncture is "complementary."

Functional Medicine is a merging of complementary medicine practices and Western medicine. Functional medicine practitioners (MDs, NDs, NPs, DCs, DOs, LAcs) are trained to treat the whole person (body, mind, and spirit) using modern medical technology, supplements, diet, IV therapy, medication, lifestyle changes and dietary enhancements. Comprehensive lab analysis is emphasized as well.

Herbalism uses plants (herbs) as remedies for medical conditions.

Holistic or Wholistic Medicine is a term used when the "whole" patient/body (as a complex system) is addressed in the wellness plan. This is in contrast to a specialist who concentrates on one particular problem or system.

Homeopathic Medicine is a practice based on a philosophy that "like cures like." A patient is treated with special homeopathic doses of a remedy that in larger amounts produce symptoms similar to those of the illness in a healthy person.

Integrative Medicine integrates complementary therapies with Western medicine to best serve the patient. The whole patient (body, mind, and spirit) is treated instead of an isolated body part.

Naturopathic Medicine (ND) is a distinct primary health care profession, emphasizing prevention, treatment, and optimal health through the use of therapeutic methods and substances that encourage the individual's inherent self-healing processes.

Osteopathic Medicine (DO) is based on structural integration (similar to chiropractic) and Western medicine, and therefore falls under the American Medical Association umbrella. Though they have their own schools, DOs must complete the same residencies as MDs, and practice very much like MDs.

Western Medicine (MD, PA, NP, RN), also known as allopathic medicine, diagnoses disease and most often treats with medications or surgery. In general practice, the whole person/body is frequently not addressed; as a result, patients are referred to specialists for each specific body part or disease state.

The lines are beginning to blur regarding who is truly offering what in healthcare. Terms such as "w/holistic" and "alternative" are sometimes used in advertising or to brand a doctor or clinic without providing detailed information about what the doctor is actually offering. For instance, you might find an MD also practicing acupuncture after studying this ancient medicine for just two hundred hours. Does that make the MD an integrated doctor? How about the chiropractor or LAc who attends two conferences on functional medicine and then markets himself as a functional medicine doctor? Or the ND who attends one minor surgery class, practices on a few patients, and then offers biopsies? It's up to you to ask your provider exactly what her education and healing philosophy are. You deserve to know this, and the practitioner should be able to answer your inquiries easily and openly.

When determining the right type of licensed healthcare professional for you, there are a few more criteria that are highly desirable. Team up with someone who:

- listens,

- sees the whole you, and

- shares knowledge (including referrals to complementary treatments) that empowers you to understand the gamut of your healthcare choices.

TEAM UP WITH A DOCTOR WHO LISTENS

Due mostly to reimbursement issues with insurance companies, many doctors do not have time to sit down with a patient and actually listen. When a doctor can engage in a conversation and delve into questions beyond "So, the nurse says you have been having chronic headaches, is that so?" magic can happen. Magic that translates into a trusting doctor/patient relationship, an understanding of what is truly happening to your body, and a general sense of well-being for both the patient and the doctor. In my practice, the first visit with a patient takes at least an hour. I need to know as much as I can about the person sitting before me. Not just what ails her, but about her life and lifestyle.

It may take some legwork, but it is essential that you take the time to find a licensed healthcare professional who listens to you intently. Why?—because the doctor who listens gleans the information needed to identify and then remove the obstacles to healing. Such a doctor will help you create and execute a comprehensive wellness plan, and not just prescribe a pharmaceutical to alleviate symptoms. The doctor who listens can offer aha moments regarding your body. Perhaps gluten is removed from your diet to address Irritable Bowel Syndrome (IBS) or you begin to walk each night and partake of a weekly massage to relieve anxiety. When your lifestyle is discussed and positive options are suggested, you have the information needed to recalibrate. You can take charge of your health.

A funny thing happens when you team up with a doctor who listens: The right questions are asked and *you* begin to tune into what your body is telling you. Chances are that with today's hectic lifestyle, you haven't heard your body screaming at you for attention. Or if you have, you've ignored it. If you learn to listen to your body and then relay that information to a doctor who is also focused on listening, you can get to the bottom of what is really happening inside.

> *A FUNNY THING HAPPENS WHEN YOU TEAM UP WITH A DOCTOR WHO LISTENS.*

CHOOSE A DOCTOR WHO SEES THE WHOLE YOU

Once you identify a healthcare professional that delights in listening and getting to know you, be sure she follows up with comprehensive, individualized care. Like naturopaths, medical doctors who are proponents of functional medicine discover the root cause of the malady, evaluate numerous labs, and see you as a whole being. Instead of addressing a specific body part or disease or illness, they see a person whose bodily systems affect one another and work together to create your overall health. They put *you* on an honest-to-goodness path to wellness. This includes collaborating on a comprehensive wellness plan that incorporates lifestyle and diet changes, supplements, and in some cases medication.

With each patient I meet, I ask this question of myself, "Is what I'm suggesting moving this person one step closer to health or to disease?" Make sure your chosen licensed healthcare professional addresses all of *you* and not just the malady that is concerning you.

CHOOSE A DOCTOR WHO SHARES

The word "doctor" is derived from the Latin for "to teach" or "to show," and if your doctor does not have time to do so, then I propose it is time to find a new one. Diagnosis followed by medication. Diagnosis—medication. Diagnosis—medication without education is not medicine; it is pharmacology at best.

BE WILLING TO NURTURE YOUR WELLNESS.

There is definitely a place for medication when treating people who are ill, but it should not be over-prescribed and alternative treatments should be proposed. Do not hesitate to ask your doctor questions in this regard. If he doesn't have an answer or know of an alternative, ask him for a referral to someone who does.

I encourage my patients to develop a healthcare team. Patients can benefit from the added skill of a chiropractor, medical doctor, or herbalist, as long as we all work together toward the common goals of healing the patient and empowering her to maintain wellness, rather than merely put up with illness.

CLARIFYING QUESTIONS TO ASK YOUR DOCTOR

- Can you offer me one or two natural options to try for three to six months before starting medication?

- I have been on medication for a long time, and I want to stop. How can you help me do this?

- Can you recommend a coach, therapist, or alternative doctor who can educate me about how to make changes to my diet and lifestyle?

- Are you willing to do more than just the standard blood tests? I like to have a more complete snapshot of my health and would like you to discuss my lab work with me in detail. My old doctor just said, "Your labs look fine."

- I have had friends and family die of cancer in the past few years. What can I do to increase my chances of preventing cancer?

- What do you think of genetic testing to learn about predisposition to disease? Do you offer it? Will you go over the results with me?

- Do you believe diet has much to do with health? It's important for me to work with a doctor who believes diet/food impacts health.

- Would you sign a petition to bar drug commercials from TV?

- What is the number one thing you would change to ensure that healthcare truly improves the health of Americans?

An adjunct to the team approach is to remember that you are the pivotal member of the team. You should ultimately be responsible for your own health. Invest in yourself and learn about the workings of your body—what it needs and what it rejects. Be willing to nurture your wellness.

NATUROPATHY AND THE HEALTH REVOLUTION

I am a proponent and practitioner of naturopathic medicine. I chose this as my profession because I believe its underlying philosophy provides a better model of care for patients.

Naturopathic doctors (NDs) are currently licensed in approximately 17 states, with each state deciding on the scope of the practice. Besides licensing in America and Canada, there is also a push by the World Naturopathic Federation to establish licensing procedures around the globe. Once this happens, naturopathic medicine will be more readily acknowledged as a healthcare alternative and will thrive in a fairer and competitive marketplace.

Naturopathic doctors offer quality time and authentic relationship to their patients in order to deliver effective care to the whole person. An average office visit with a ND lasts about forty-five minutes, the time needed to explore the cause of the ailment, which is unique to the patient, and to discuss tailored treatment options. We search for the reason why a person is sick. When I see a patient for the first time, I interview him to determine what the symptoms are, what kind of lifestyle, habits, and hobbies he engages in, and most importantly, what he is willing to do to change his health. I endeavor to get a whole picture of the whole person and how he relates to life.

A patient once shared with me that her medical doctor said her digestive distress (bloating, diarrhea, and constipation) had nothing to do with stress. How could this woman's emotions regarding the recent death of her mother, a divorce, and incessant insomnia have nothing to do with her digestion? A person's body, emotions, and life's concerns are all connected. That is a foundational belief of naturopathic medicine. Stress is absolutely related to this person's acute digestive issues. Instead of prescribing an antacid and telling her "not to worry," I offered this patient real solutions to real problems: assistance from a weekly grief group, comprehensive lab work, digestive enzymes taken with meals, a calming bath two times a week, and biking or walking with friends after work. When this woman embraced these suggestions, within ten days she reported that she felt 90 percent better. Her integrated wellness plan not only helped her heal physically but also encouraged her to be more engaged with life. She took matters in her own hands and began to see a therapist to find relief regarding her divorce and mother's death. The antacid prescribed by the MD would never have gotten to the root cause of her discomfort nor would it have helped heal this woman's grief. She, like so many of us, needed to be heard and attended to as a whole person.

Most of us desire to feel good, enjoy our lives, and live disease free. It is my belief that naturopathic medicine can help many of us meet these goals. Achieving good health does not need to be complicated, but one must be courageous and committed to investing time and energy into the endeavor.

CHAPTER 2 HEALTH RESOLUTION

Think about the healthcare professionals you currently have in your life. Are you satisfied? Dissatisfied? Maybe you do not even have someone to turn to.

Let's change that. Can you make a pledge to find at least one doctor or licensed, integrative healthcare practitioner who listens to you, sees you, and teaches you? Give yourself a deadline. Do what it takes to invest in one of the most important things in your life—your whole-self health.

"I, _____, commit to finding at least one licensed healthcare practitioner to help me with my _____.
I will make an appointment by this date _____."

CHAPTER 3

The Foundation of Naturopathic Medicine

Do you remember the last time you had a paper cut on your hand? Ouch, right? Did you take a moment and wonder how your body actually healed itself from this small, yet bothersome wound? And so quickly!

This body-healing-itself phenomenon is part of the invisible, mysterious force naturopathic doctors call "the healing power of nature," "life force," or "internal healing." We naturopathic doctors practice medicine based on the principle attributed to Hippocrates called *Vis Medicatrix Naturae*, which translates into "the healing power of nature." In the same way a forest heals itself from the devastation of a fire because of *Vis Medicatrix Naturae*, or as I like to call it, *The Vis*, the human body, which is part of nature, has the innate ability to heal itself from infections, injuries, and chronic disease. The heart of naturopathic medicine is the belief that we have within us the power to heal ourselves with a little help from our friends—diet, clean environment, movement, knowledge of how the body works, and when necessary, supplementation, medication, and surgery.

The entire natural world strives to live in equilibrium and harmony—and that includes us humans. Consider this: If you should cut your arm quite deeply, it will not be the stitches and antibiotics that heal your wound. Although they certainly help, they're just synthetic catgut and chemicals. Then what is the catalyst to the actual knitting of the cut—the healing? How does the body know to expel foreign debris from the wound? How does it know to grow new skin? It is this "consciousness," this "hidden power," that scientists and theologians continually attempt to decipher. It will be a long time before we figure this out, if ever. It's the mystery of life, and it's this mystery that healers must trust before true healing, not just the suppression of symptoms, can occur. Doctors need to trust in a higher power: nature, *The Vis*, *chi*, the innate, or love, for true healing to begin. Unfortunately, many doctors have forgotten the body has a built-in ability to heal; therefore patients are not taught this. Until this issue is dealt with in Western medicine, our current medical healthcare system will fail the people. It will make lots of people in the field of medicine financially rich and the patient medically poor.

> MANY DOCTORS HAVE FORGOTTEN THE BODY HAS A BUILT-IN ABILITY TO HEAL.

Nature has its laws, and my main job and responsibility as a naturopathic doctor is to trust, practice, and espouse these laws. I would not plant a watermelon seed, deprive it of sun, water, and love and expect it to grow. So why would I expect a patient to be in a state of health if they get four hours of sleep a night, eat processed foods, and drink coffee and soda throughout the day? There's a natural order to follow, and if we choose not to do so, we won't be our healthiest. Yes, there are always those who argue, "My grandpa never let water pass his lips, ate bacon, and drank whiskey his whole life, and lived to be 95." Lucky duck! Some people do live outside the normal bell curve of nature and science. I am not going to gamble that I am one of them. Also, how did Grandpa feel each and every day? That is the question and may be the reason he drank that whiskey.

I was introduced to and fascinated by the philosophy of *Vis Medicatrix Naturae* while studying at Southwest College of Naturopathic Medicine in Tempe, Arizona. Today, I still look at disease through the lenses of *The Vis* and am in awe of nature's practicality and efficiency. Take, for example, a fever. When a virus or bacteria has upset the body's natural balance, the body's response is a fever (*The Vis*), thus creating an environment in which the bacteria or virus cannot survive. Often it is just fine to let a fever run its course while remaining hydrated, resting, taking certain botanical herbs, and closely monitoring the situation. Fever is a form of healing and not necessarily something to reduce.

Another example of *The Vis* that many people can relate to is allergies. The body sneezes and discharges mucous out of the nose and eyes in an attempt to rid itself of the allergens causing the reaction. Most of the time, we resort to over-the-counter medications to hide and suppress these symptoms. Suppressing symptoms does not cure allergies. Taking time to understand the imbalance within the body's systems, determining the reason for the response, and building the immune system to prevent the allergic response from occurring again will *eliminate* allergies.

Many of us can also relate to stomach upsets or food poisoning. Who has escaped the pleasure of bowing to the porcelain god for 12 to 24 hours in between sitting on it? Again, these unpleasant reactions of vomiting and diarrhea are the body's innate effort to restore homeostasis to the organism (the human) by expelling the toxins being released by the microorganism causing the distress. In this case, the last thing you want to do is to stop the vomiting or diarrhea. This is the body functioning well. Instead of downing anti-diarrheal or anti-emetic medications, focus on resting, staying hydrated, and catching up on old episodes of *Seinfeld*, *Saturday Night Live*, or another favorite series. Remind yourself that this, too, shall pass and trust that your body knows best.

The philosophy of naturopathic medicine is to work with the body's innate wisdom in a powerful and synergistic way, rather than to suppress the natural healing power within us/our bodies. This has been the goal of naturopathic doctors for over a century. Naturopathy is not a New Age fad; it is a tried and true healing practice. NDs have been practicing for over 100 years in the United States, long before the modern day pharmacy drive-through.

EARLY NATUROPATHY IN AMERICA

Have you ever eaten Fruit Loops, Corn Flakes, or a Pop-Tart for breakfast? If you answered "yes," then you have partaken in naturopathic history. Brothers Will and Dr. John Harvey Kellogg were established businessmen in the natural food industry in the late 1800s and were leading the way to healthy living in America after studying with practitioners in Europe. In the early 1900s, however, Dr. John Harvey and Will developed a difference of opinion concerning the direction of their young company. Will wanted to add sugar to their newly invented cereal because he thought it would increase sales. Dr. John Harvey, an early naturopathic doctor, was adamant that they stick to unsweetened whole grain. Sugar separated the two brothers (who never spoke again) and their beloved company. It's ironic that the Kellogg brothers' early search for healthier living led to a processed food super giant. And also sad, given that 17 percent of children and more than 30 percent of adults are considered obese in the United

States today, with sugar being a leading contributor to this disease.[1]

The Kellogg brothers were initially influenced by the work of Father Sebastian Kneipp, a Catholic priest in Germany. In the mid to late 1800s, Father Kneipp was renowned as a healer who cured diseases naturally, without medication, and also as the father of hydrotherapy. Hydrotherapy embraces the use of water in a variety of ways to help cure medical maladies. It includes such actions as drinking pure water, sitz baths, enemas, and soaking in hot springs. People from around the globe and all walks of life flocked to study with Dr. Kneipp and be healed by his medical secrets and "nature cure."

Dr. John Harvey Kellogg was one of Father Kneipp's students, and he spent months learning Father Kneipp's treatment methods based on *Vis Medicatrix Naturae*. Enthused by all he had learned, Dr. Kellogg returned to the United States, and opened his famous sanatorium in Battle Creek, Michigan, helping patients heal from many diseases using hydrotherapy, whole grain foods, rest, and sunshine. He also wrote *Rational Hydrotherapy*, first published in 1901, which remains one of the most definitive textbooks on hydrotherapy and is still taught in naturopathic medical school. If you live in San Diego, Seattle, Portland, Chicago, or Bridgeport, Connecticut, you are

---

1. "The State of Obesity 2015: Better Policies for a Healthier America," Robert Wood Johnson Foundation, Trust for America's Health, www.healthyamericans.org, accessed November 24, 2015, http://stateofobesity.org/files/stateofobesity2015.pdf.

lucky because last time I checked, the naturopathic medical schools in these cities still offer these rare, effective, and restorative treatments.

Around the turn of the century, another American, Henry Lindlahr also consulted Father Kneipp. Lindlahr had been unable to find relief from his diabetes and obesity through Western medicine. (Americans were already struggling with diabetes and obesity 100 years ago and seeking help outside the traditional medical system.) Upon returning to the United States 40 pounds lighter and no longer diabetic, he enrolled in the Homeopathic and Eclectic College of Illinois, and after graduating in 1904, he opened the Lindlahr Sanatorium in Chicago. Dr. Lindlahr practiced Father Kneipp's hydrotherapy along with breathwork, fasting, cleanses, specialized diet, exercise, rest, sunlight, talk therapy, and fever therapy (inducing a high fever in order to jump-start the immune system to kill unwanted bacteria, viruses, and cancers). His early 20th century sanatorium shared much in common with our integrated medical centers today. Unfortunately, such centers are few and far between and patients must often travel hundreds of miles to access them in order to recover from illness while adopting a healthier lifestyle.

Henry Lindlahr also founded the Lindlahr College of Natural Therapeutics, which became the leading naturopathic college of the day. In 1913, he wrote *Nature Cure*, a must read for anyone interested in the history of all medical practice in America, not just naturopathy.

Another pioneer of naturopathic medicine was also a student and patient of Father Kneipp—Dr. Benedict Lust (pronounced Loost). Dr. Lust was born in Germany and immigrated to the United States. When he contracted tuberculosis and American doctors were unable to help him, he returned to Germany seeking Father Kneipp's cure. Successfully healed from tuberculosis, Dr. Lust returned back to United States and graduated from the New York Homeopathic Medical College. He became known as the "father of naturopathic medicine," practicing and teaching Father Kneipp's methodology and naturopathic medicine until his death in the 1940s. Among his accomplishments was the founding of his "healthcare store." At this store, one could buy whole grains, homeopathic remedies, herbal tinctures, and books on healing techniques from around the world. Today, if you shop at a natural food store, you have Dr. Lust and naturopathic medicine to thank for the very existence of this type of establishment.

Upon graduating from naturopathic school in 2004, I, too, opened a natural foods store in Mancos, Colorado, with two wonderful co-partners. Our mission was to provide a place within our community where ideas could be exchanged, education could occur, and health-related books could be purchased. And, of course, you could buy natural foods and medicines. Today, Zuma Natural Foods remains a hub in this flourishing rural community. I thank Dr. Lust for setting an example and creating the prototype. It's nice knowing that your neighbors have a stepping-stone as they journey closer to wellness and away from disease.

THE CRUX OF NATUROPATHY

Father Kneipp, Dr. John Harvey Kellogg, Dr. Lindlahr, and Dr. Lust were the pioneers of what has become today's practice of American naturopathic medicine. Its purpose is to empower individuals to heal themselves of illness and disease by working with the power of nature. To be either a doctor or a patient of naturopathic medicine you must BELIEVE in *The Vis*—the inimitable healing ability of nature.

In his book *Philosophy of Natural Therapeutics*, Dr. Henry Lindlahr states that the primary cause of all disease is violation of nature's laws.[2] Though his wording is somewhat outdated, I believe we can all relate his philosophy to our modern lifestyles. In chapter five of *Philosophy of Natural Therapeutics*, he states that disease is rooted in three main causes. Essentially, he asserts that all disease is caused by:

- *Low vitality and low energy from doing too much of everything.* Doesn't this sound familiar? Seventy-five percent of my patients say they have low energy, but continue to go, go, go.

- *Abnormal blood and lymph function due to eating food low in nutrients, especially lacking in mineral salts.* This can be summed up as eating too many

2. Henry Lindlahr, *Philosophy of Natural Therapeutics* (Essex, England: The C.W. Daniel Company Limited, 1975) 19.

processed foods and not enough nutrient-dense foods such as fruits, vegetables, and proteins.

- *Accumulation of waste material in the body.* This is why naturopathic doctors stress the importance of one to two healthy bowel movements a day, drinking lots of water, and engaging in daily exercise to flush toxins out of the body.

The crux of what naturopathic medicine confronts today is that people have drifted too far away from nature. We have interrupted natural rhythms and bodily cycles, natural foods, and natural ways of healing. It is time to return to what actually nourishes and heals us, and if I am hearing correctly, it's what many patients want their healthcare to include.

THE NATUROPATHIC THERAPEUTIC ORDER

Throughout the twentieth century, public interest in naturopathy swayed in the United States. There were times when the practice nearly perished and others when it flourished. Over the years, NDs have had the time to collaborate, work, study, and codify what it means to be a naturopath.

When working with patients, naturopathic doctors follow a systematic therapeutic order, or hierarchy, of healing based on the findings of our ND predecessors. We approach each individual's health with fresh eyes and an open mind. We listen, ask questions, develop hypotheses as to what might be the issue or issues for the patient and then create a wellness plan following this therapeutic order. Our basic goal is to build the patient's health from the bottom up, and that begins with a sound foundation.

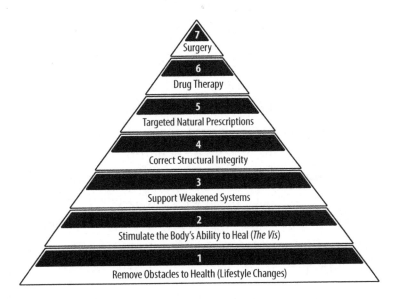

The Naturopathic Therapeutic Order

(The order of treatment received by a patient may vary depending upon immediate health-related needs and the particular ND practice.)

The Naturopathic Therapeutic Order, first crafted by Jared Zeff, ND, LAc, and Pamela Snider, ND, offers an order of actions to take when creating a wellness plan for a patient. It begins with the gentlest, practical actions and only when it is absolutely necessary employs drug therapy and surgery—Western medical practices. Here is how I utilize the Naturopathic Therapeutic Order in my practice:

1. A healthy foundation is built by removing obstacles to health. This is most often manifested by

adjustment to lifestyle, such as dietary changes, sleep hygiene, and exercise. Labs are often ordered to provide information needed to suggest proper care.

2. While building a healthy foundation, naturopathic doctors will stimulate the innate healing ability that exists in every patient—*The Vis*. This divine force is activated by introducing therapies that aid healing the whole self. Therapies might include acupuncture, acupressure, physical therapy, hydrotherapy, the prescribing of nutritional supplements (supplementation), and meditation, among others. Auxiliary therapies, such as talk therapy, art therapy, or music therapy, may also be recommended to provide emotional and spiritual support to the patient.

3. Additional support is provided to specific systems of the body (digestive, skeletal, circulatory/respiratory, immune, and nervous) needing attention. For example, the immune and respiratory systems would be targeted for extra assistance in a patient with chronic allergies. This may entail supplementation and the continuation of therapies recommended in phase two.

4. Once the bodily systems and organs are reinforced, physical medicine such as chiropractic or massage is used to obtain structural alignment. In many cases, this would be a continuation of treatments initiated in tiers two and three.

5. NDs commonly employ natural nutritional supplements to control and ease symptoms while searching for the more fundamental cause of an imbalance. These would include vitamins, minerals, herbs, homeopathic remedies, and natural food supplements. I might put together a botanical tincture to aid digestion while testing a patient for food allergies, or offer a vitamin supplement to fend off an acute head cold and boost the immune system, or deliver nutritional IV therapy for a chronic illness. Though symptom management is not ideal, it is necessary in cases where symptoms are so unpleasant and chronic that immediate relief is a priority. Supplementation is very often included in the second tier of the therapeutic order, as well, to assist the body in healing itself. Supplements become part of the wellness plan at various points, depending on the patient's condition and the ND's approach.

This fifth tier in the therapeutic order illustrates the way the public most readily construes naturopathy. New patients to my practice will immediately ask, "What can I take for a headache?" "Is there something natural for back pain?" "What can I do about this bloating?" There is no one to blame for this misperception but the naturopathic profession. Offering a supplement to "fix" something is akin to an MD prescribing a medication. I feel obligated to remind both patients and colleagues that we mustn't jump to this later treatment step. It is much more prudent to follow the first steps of the order and shift lifestyle, educate, and empower patients before offering supplements or the next level on the therapeutic order—drug therapy.

6. In states where it is legal, a naturopathic doctor might prescribe medications if the earlier tiered treatments are not moving the patient closer to health. If the ND cannot prescribe medications, the patient can be referred to a trusted medical doctor, one that sees the ND as a team member in achieving your health goals and not as a competitor.

7. The last tier on the therapeutic order is to accept procedures by medical specialists. At this stage, patients have a disease that has progressed enough to warrant more invasive interventions, such as surgery, radiation, and chemotherapy. When a patient's condition justifies these treatments, usually in a life-or-death situation, naturopathic treatments can still be a part of the plan. I often work with people both pre- and post-surgery to bolster the body and to help it heal as quickly as possible. Integrated oncology is another great example of this. The MD oncologist focuses on the chemo and radiation therapies while the ND oncologist focuses on restoring overall health and prevention of potential acute issues such as infection, which could set back treatment and healing.

The Naturopathic Therapeutic Order provides NDs with a set protocol. It is essential to understand, nonetheless, that the immediate needs of the patient take precedent over the order. If a new patient comes into the office experiencing acute symptoms indicating a possible heart attack, discussing lifestyle changes isn't appropriate or responsible. Surgery, the seventh tier of the therapeutic order, might be. It all comes down to truly listening to the patient's concerns in order to understand what is going on. The ND ascertains the patient's perspective regarding the state of the patient's health, and then investigates further to determine the source of the issue. The therapeutic order provides a framework from which to develop an orderly approach to treatment.

Naturopathic doctors and *The Vis* have a critical role to play in The Health Revolution and the future of healthcare. Author Mark Hyman, MD, who is a leader in the functional medicine movement said, "The origins of functional medicine stretch back into the history of naturopathic medicine—on the idea that health is not the absence of disease, but the creation of vitality and abundant health. Many of the principles of naturopathic medicine—the body as a self-organizing, self-healing dynamic system, the concepts of detoxification and digestive health, and food as medicine are all now embedded with Functional Medicine."

Change is in the air regarding how we approach our healthcare. Each of us, as consumer and as human, has the right to choose the type of care we feel works best for our whole selves. There's a place for all—alternative, functional, naturopathic, and Western medicine. Let's work together and all become healthy.

———

CHAPTER 3 HEALTH RESOLUTION

Nature heals. My years working in a wilderness therapy program have allowed me to witness this fact firsthand. When was the last time you spent time in the outdoors? Even if you live in the city, nature is accessible in a park or oftentimes after an hour-long road trip. For your overall health, I encourage you to set aside time weekly to spend at least one hour in nature. Walk barefoot in the grass. Lie on your back and look at the sunlight filter through the tree canopy. Camp out and enjoy the color, pop, and smoky scent of a fire. Gift yourself moments of silence when you are in this natural chapel. Set aside enough time to reflect, meditate, and absorb the medicine that comes from Mother Earth.

On this day, _____ , I will go to

_____

and heal in nature.

CHAPTER 4

Guidelines for Optimum Health

Licensed medical doctors (MDs) and Doctors of Osteopathy (DOs) are trained in the practice of diagnosis, treatment, and the prevention of disease, but the art of healing is not unique to them. Healing is accessible to each and every one of us. Healing comes from within, supported by nature, our food, community, and love.

If we are given the education, tools, and understanding that over time our bodies can heal themselves, we can all ultimately enjoy optimum health. We can be an integral force in our very own healing. Just like a forest recovers from a fire, we can become rejuvenated and more robust than ever before.

The intention with this book is to educate and empower you so that you can successfully collaborate with your healthcare team. I've boiled down my education, years in practice, patient successes, and my own quest for a dynamic life into eight guidelines for achieving and maintaining ideal health and longevity. These are as follows:

- Hydrate

- Eat real food

- Supplement wisely

- Balance hormones

- Learn from labs

- De-stress

- Create community

- Move your body

The following chapters will cover each guideline in more depth, but a short synopsis is provided here.

HYDRATE

The old adage is true. If you're thirsty, you're already dehydrated. Listen to your body if it says, "Water me," and take action. Drink pure, filtered, delicious water.

Proper hydration means you consume adequate amounts of filtered water daily, which varies per the individual. A rough guideline is to drink half your weight in ounces. For example, a 150-pound person would drink 75 ounces of water each day.

Water fuels cells, allows for clear communication between cells, and flushes out waste products via urination and bowel movements. Don't stagnate; keep the body running clean and pure with water. The bonus: hydration can make you look five years younger. So, cheers!

EAT REAL FOOD

Eating real food seems so simple, and yet it's the biggest hurdle for many of us. There are constant temptations, and often it's just plain difficult to find real food. Ever drive down one of those fast food alleys when you're starving? It's hell!

We need to avoid those brilliant marketing strategies and empty calories the food industry likes to dangle before us, and instead buy local, organic, non-GMO food over everything else. Nutrient-dense foods provide the body and brain with key ingredients to function at optimal levels. Eat fresh vegetables, fruits, meat, nuts, seeds, broths, and other whole foods that provide the body with necessary vitamins, minerals, and nutrients, as well as vitality.

SUPPLEMENT WISELY

Supplements can be very effective when taken with prevention and support in mind. They can build and assist bodily systems for ultimate functioning. For example, probiotics boost gut health, zinc bolsters the immune system, and essential fatty acids provide much-needed omega 3s for brain health.

Please don't lean heavily on supplements to achieve the best possible health. As with medications, keep supplements to a minimum, and regularly review why and if it is still beneficial to take a given supplement.

BALANCE HORMONES

If your hormones are not in balance, then it's quite likely you are not in balance. Insulin, estrogen, thyroid stimulating hormone (TSH), testosterone, and vitamin D are all examples of hormones we want to maintain at favorable levels. Hormones direct our moods, fertility, blood sugar, weight management, sleep, and so much more. Balanced hormones = a happier, healthier you.

LEARN FROM LABS

Laboratory tests vary greatly in the way samples are taken and what they determine. Such tests include but aren't limited to blood draws, urine and stool samples, saliva samples, radiology tests such as MRIs, ultrasound and CAT scans, throat swabs, and EKGs. You can even have your genetics tested by companies online.

Lab test results offer both the patient and the doctor information that can help determine where the body is functioning well and where it needs nourishment and support. Once labs provide objective insight defining the status of a bodily system or organ, the information gleaned can direct treatment that will build a foundation of wellness.

DE-STRESS

As our lives become busier and busier, and we are bombarded by technology, news, and worry, it becomes ever more important to unwind and become centered. Proper rest and "unplugging" from day-to-day routines and stimuli are part of a foundational wellness plan.

In order to successfully de-stress, take the time to jump off the hamster wheel and discover a form of relaxation that resonates with you. As a doctor, I am quite often giving patients an open prescription to stop and smell the roses.

CREATE COMMUNITY

Living, working, and playing in a caring and thriving community are often overlooked when devising a wellness plan. Excellent health is contagious and the more you align with people who confirm a positive lifestyle, the more likely you are to have a vibrant, healthy life. Find your

EXCELLENT HEALTH IS CONTAGIOUS.

people and/or animals, share your love for life, be of service, and become active in your community in a way that gives back to you and to others.

MOVE YOUR BODY

Movement of the body promotes good health. There is no shortage of wonderful ways to get the muscles moving and to send oxygen all the way through to your fingers and toes. Jump-start this goal by doing what sounds totally engaging or what you have always dreamed of doing—from walking the dogs in the rain, working out at a community gym, to entering a triathlon.

There's an added benefit to movement: it often destresses, so you achieve two health benefits from the effort of one action.

CONNECTING TO SOMETHING BIGGER

My eight guidelines fall under an umbrella concept that is forever useful while on a quest for excellent health: It is the idea of connecting to something greater than yourself and trusting in a higher power. This idea can be off-putting to some and even scary, but I would be remiss not to introduce it.

Consider this: What or whom can you trust?

There are an infinite number of answers to this question. You may trust your partner, your cat, or WebMD®, but what about the bigger things in which you can trust such as God and love? Have you felt the power of love for someone or something? Then you know how it can literally make the cells in your body dance. Trust love. Take it and give it each and every day, not just on Valentine's Day.

And how about the power of nature? Many individuals feel at peace and a sense of belonging when they are in the wilderness. I find that I am in awe of the ecosystems and the grandeur of it all. Why not allow yourself to be part of that? Trust nature's awe-some-ness every day, and not only on a vacation to the beach or Yellowstone.

I would like to share an experience I had with a dear friend that forever altered my understanding of connection to something larger than myself. In the year 2000, my friend's two-year-old nephew died of unknown causes. Upon hearing this news, my friend and I, who were living in Hawaii at the time, walked to the beach to offer prayers and swim in the warm, healing water. We prayed and cried.

What was it like to be in my friend's shoes? I wondered. How was she dealing with the anger, grief, and remorse? How would she cope? I looked to the sky for answers. As I blinked away tears, I watched wispy white clouds grow against a backdrop of blue. They floated into a pattern. They wrote a word in the sky: "Leo." Was I seeing things? And what did it mean? Her nephew wasn't named Leo.

I turned to my friend and asked, "Was your nephew a Leo? I mean, when was his birthday?"

"July," she said. "Why do you ask?"

As more tears flowed, I pointed to the heavens. She saw the word "Leo" immediately, so I wasn't imagining it. Leo was her nephew's astrological sign. We watched in awe as "Leo" hovered above for a good five minutes. In that time, a sense of comfort, belonging, and trust in the divine swept over our bodies, and I knew there was a spirit of nature, God—something—much more powerful than I. This memory is forever stamped on my existence, for when I doubt, I think back to Leo in the sky.

Health is not just about an annual exam and labs that may suggest a need for medication. Health is about being part of a living tapestry. It's about believing you are powerful as part of something truly magnificent. The benefit you receive from this trust is a more dynamic you, vibrating at a higher level of consciousness, and with the ability to offer the world your gifts. We all have a purpose, and it's often our duty to dig a little deeper to discover it. Then we get to reap the rewards of sharing that purpose—our bliss— with the world.

HEALTH IS ABOUT BEING PART OF A LIVING TAPESTRY.

The belief that we are part of something larger than ourselves is at the center of my wellness plans. I nudge patients to become connected, whether to their own version of God, a spiritually oriented organization, meditation, yoga, nature, or whatever makes sense for them. We are a very small part of something much greater, and there is power in surrendering to this truth.

CHAPTER 4 HEALTH RESOLUTION

Do you have a Leo in the sky? Is there something or someone in this universe in which you can trust and from which you can gain solace? Some of us find such comfort in a 12-step program, working in a soup kitchen, gardening, attending a church, temple, or shrine, hiking the backcountry, or following a coach or mentor. If you haven't considered this possibility, give it a moment of your time. Write down three possible places, people, or ideas that may connect you to something bigger than yourself. There is something out there for each of us.

1. _____

2. _____

3. _____

CHAPTER 5

Life Water

By the time we're in first grade, most of us recognize the molecular formula H_2O—water. Water is the foundation for life on Earth, and the master elixir for living vibrantly day to day.

Water is not an endless resource though, despite the fact that we treat it as such. It's time to think twice about taking long showers, watering never-used lawns, and running water down the drain while brushing our teeth. As I write this book, the state of California is experiencing one of the worst droughts in history. Many municipalities are at long last imposing water conservation measures, though we have known and predicted this scenario for a number of years.

When the well is run dry, we will realize
the value of water. —Ben Franklin

As we begin The Health Revolution, the time is right to become more aware of and creative around water conservation. It is time to expand our vision of this precious commodity so future generations have enough *clean* water to survive.

Water on Earth is like the blood in our veins; without it there is no life.

THE GIFT OF HYDRATION

Drinking adequate amounts of clean water is necessary to obtain and maintain excellent health. Water hydrates the body and is the catalyst for the elimination of waste through tears, sweating, urination, and bowel movements. As you may recall, both Dr. Henry Lindlahr and Dr. John Harvey Kellogg used hydrotherapy in treating patients as naturopathy began in America. It is still a valid and healing practice used today, and it is based on good old H_2O.

Enjoying 10 to 20 ounces of water is a fantastic way to start your day, but don't stop there. To remain hydrated, 50 percent of one's body weight (in ounces) of water is the suggested daily intake. For example, a 200-pound person would drink 100 ounces (ten 10-ounce glasses) of water each day. Most of us consume less than 20 percent of our body weight, resulting in dehydration. This prompts common complaints such as constipation, depression, fatigue, headaches, dry and itchy skin, and a general lack of vitality. For some, dehydration can lead to elevated blood pressure.

Many Americans drink more soda than water. A recent national Gallup poll found that half of Americans drink one or more glasses of soda a day, with seven percent saying they drink four or more sodas daily.[1] Imagine the money we could all save and the health we could gain just by convincing folks to switch from soda to good old-fashioned water.

An example of water to the rescue lies with a 54-year-old patient of mine who had high blood pressure, high cholesterol, and chronic pain. He reduced his medications by 75 percent in just two months by instilling a few of my health tenets into his lifestyle. One of these was increasing his daily water consumption from eight ounces a day to 90 and decreasing his soda consumption from four a day to one. Not only did his bodily systems find restored balance, but he also lost 18 pounds, was in significantly less pain, felt energetic, began playing tennis again, and became hopeful about his future.

DO OTHER BEVERAGES COUNT AS WATER?

Most clients ask me what counts as water towards their "half their body weight in ounces." I keep it simple: water, water with fresh lemon or lime added to it, and truly herbal teas (not decaffeinated teas), all without added sugar or

1. Lydia Saad, "Nearly Half of Americans Drink Soda Daily," Gallup.com, Well-Being, July 23, 2012, last accessed January 27, 2016, http://www.gallup.com/poll/156116/nearly-half-americans-drink-soda-daily.aspx.

cream. Coffee, caffeinated tea, soda, carbonated water, any type of juice, sports and energy drinks, and all those fancy bottled waters with additives and marketing gimmicks surrounding them do not count as water.

THE FILTER AND CONTAINER COUNT

The best water to drink is filtered and from a glass or stainless steel container. No plastic, please. Chemicals from the plastic can leach into the water and disrupt bodily systems, especially the endocrine and nervous systems, preventing them from proper functioning. Biologists, zoologists, and chemists are publishing volumes of research on the detrimental effects plastics have on our bodies and on the environment. I say, "Better safe than sorry," since the shift from plastic to stainless steel or glass containers is easier now than ever before. For more information on this topic, see Mariah Blake's article in *Mother Jones* called "The Scary New Evidence on BPA-Free Plastics and the Big Tobacco-style Campaign to Bury It."[2] It's certainly worth the read, as it shares research proving that the plastic sippy cups so many American children drink from daily leach synthetic estrogens into the contents. An imbalance of estrogen, especially synthetic, can affect bone growth, ovulation, and heart function. Like I said, "Better safe than sorry!"

2. Mariah Blake, "The Scary New Evidence on BPA-Free Plastics and the Big Tobacco-style Campaign to Bury It," *Mother Jones*, accessed June 6, 2016, http://www.motherjones.com/environment/2014/03/tritan-certichem-eastman-bpa-free-plastic-safe.

Filters help rid water of lead, chloride, fluoride, pharmaceutical remnants, and other contaminants found in today's water supplies. Do you know what is in your water? Call your local municipality and see what filtration system they have in place and what they add to your water in the name of public safety. Perhaps we all should hold municipalities responsible for supplying pure, filtered drinking water to all. There are governmental agencies, plumbers, and other third parties who will test your water for a range of impurities. You can even go to Culligan.com/home/water-testing and schedule a free basic water test in your home. Investing in a home water filtration system is a great way to jump-start better health. Any filtration is better than none. Prices for filtration systems range from thirty dollars to thousands of dollars. It might take some effort, but it's worth finding one that meets your health and financial needs.

I use a small countertop water filtration system from New Wave Enviro Products that is easily installed on most kitchen faucets within minutes. It costs about 100 dollars, and a replacement filter is needed every 10 to 14 months, which runs about 85 dollars. I like this model because it's easy to install, minimizes many impurities, and the tap water tastes noticeably fresher.

If you have ample space, you may consider a larger counter top stainless steel filter. This type of system often catches more impurities than the one I currently use. The drawbacks to this type of system are the space it takes, the fact that you must manually pour water into the cistern, and the cost, which is typically two to three times more than a faucet model.

Whole-house filtration systems and those installed beneath the sink are fantastic options, albeit a bit pricey. If you own your home, this is a healthful choice to make when you are investing in improvements or desire a worthwhile do-it-yourself project.

The point is to start somewhere regarding filtering your water. Purchase a water filtration system that works for you, your family, your home, and your budget. Your body will thank you and the water will taste fresher, which may get you drinking more of this essential life source.

SPRING WATER

Some of the best water available comes from fresh mountain or sea level springs. Have you ever been driving down a scenic road and wondered why people were parking their cars and stepping out with glass jars and jugs? Inevitably, they know of a natural spring where they can harvest delicious water. Spring water is usually unadulterated with chemicals, although I advise you to check with locals in the know to make sure you can drink the water without treating it or boiling it. If you would like to find a natural spring near you, check out Findaspring.com.

HOT SPRINGS & BATHS

The world is blessed with healing hot springs. For thousands of years people have relied on hot springs to rejuvenate their spirits, heal injuries and sore muscles, and soothe chronic aches and pains. Whether it's the healing minerals found in hot springs that promote relaxation or the heat of the water, or both, people across the globe and over many centuries attest to their healing attributes. A few of my favorite American hot springs are Esalen in California, Avalanche Ranch, Orvis, and Trimble Hot Springs in Colorado, Olympic National Park in Washington, Ahalanui Park in Hawaii, and a few remote springs in Death Valley, California.

If visiting natural hot springs is not an option for you, many pools and spas now use salt water or copper systems instead of chlorine. This makes pools and hot tubs more attractive and therapeutic without all those smelly chemicals.

You can also create a hot springs effect in your own home by soaking in a very warm bath (98° to 102° Fahrenheit) with added Epsom salt and a favorite essential oil. Close your eyes and imagine yourself in the vastness of nature soaking under the stars. Baths such as this induce relaxation, decrease inflammation, treat dry skin and rashes, and sooth tight and over-used muscles. I often prescribe taking a warm, candlelit bath an hour before bed to patients suffering from insomnia. If you are brave enough, end the warm bath with a cool to cold shower. Though it will feel invigorating in the moment, my patients report that a cool shower actually helps them sleep soundly throughout the night.

HYDRATION AND BOWEL MOVEMENTS

Naturopathic doctors are not shy when it comes to asking about bowel movements. Your pooping schedule tells us a lot about your body chemistry and state of health. I find that most new patients need help increasing the frequency of bowel movements. Ideally, you should have one to three bowel movements a day. Over half the people I treat have three to four bowel movements a week. That's just not enough.

I remember a case study from medical school. A patient had gone to her family doctor, and lab results indicated that the patient had high levels of cholesterol, triglycerides, and thyroid-stimulating hormone. The doctor wanted to put her on two medications to address the abnormal labs. This patient did not want to start medication, so she came to our naturopathic clinic looking for alternatives. While interviewing her, I asked how often she had a bowel movement, and she said, "Two times."

I reported this to the head doctor. He looked at me and asked, "Two times a day or a week?"

I thought he was crazy for asking that question, but I honored his request to obtain clarification from the patient.

To my surprise, she said, "Two times a week." I thought for sure she had meant two times a day. But to her, two times a week was normal. It had never been any other way.

We designed a wellness plan that included (but was not limited to) a commitment to drinking at least 60 ounces of water a day, eating more whole foods instead of processed foods, exercising, and consistently taking a few warranted supplements. Within six weeks she was having daily bowel movements, not two weekly. Within a few months she'd lost weight, was rid of her chronic joint pain, her hair was no longer falling out, and her libido returned full force, much to her delight. She never started medication, and her lab work returned to more normal ranges. During her last office visit, she shared that she had booked a plane ticket to Europe to visit her sister whom she hadn't seen in 20 years. She was not only healed, she was invigorated!

Daily bowel movements should be a priority. We eliminate bodily waste through sweat, urine, and excrement. If we don't sweat daily, then most of us rely on urination and bowel movements to get the job done. A significant cause of disease is insufficient elimination of waste from the body; therefore, pooping is essential for better health. Daily bowel movements not only help you feel more energetic and less bloated and sluggish, they may also decrease your risk of colon cancer, hemorrhoids, and other inflammatory digestive issues such as SIBO (Small Intestine Bacterial Overgrowth), IBS (Irritable Bowel Syndrome), IBD (Inflammatory Bowel Disease), and GERD (Gastroesophageal Reflux Disease). Lastly, bowel movements are 75 percent water.

The remainder consists of fiber, bacteria, mucous, and other sloughed cells. Remaining hydrated is necessary for daily, healthy bowel movements. So cheers to drinking more water and providing for your daily movement.

The key to healthy bowel movements is a healthy gut. I like to tell patients to "treat their guts as prime real estate." Hydrating, eating real food (which we'll cover in the next chapter), and movement of the body assist in this goal. Drinking ten ounces of water with or without the juice of half a fresh lemon in the morning can work as a natural laxative. If you change your gut, you can change your life, and that might begin with a very humble start, such as pooping every day.

> *I LIKE TO TELL PATIENTS TO "TREAT THEIR GUTS AS PRIME REAL ESTATE."*

HYDROTHERAPY

Hydrotherapy utilizes water in a variety of ways to treat many medical ailments. Drinking adequate amounts of water is hydrotherapy in its simplest form. A few other options are sitz baths, bathing in hot springs, enemas, walking barefoot on the morning dew, snow walking, and the "grandfather of them all:" constitutional hydrotherapy. Constitutional hydrotherapy treatments consist of alternating applications of hot and cold towels to the abdomen and back, along with very gentle electrical stimulation to the spine that aids in detoxification by stimulating the organs of digestion and elimination.

Hydrotherapy takes advantage of the physical properties of water, such as temperature and pressure, to stimulate circulation of blood and lymph. If a patient has a sore throat for example, a ND might suggest he wrap a very warm compress around his neck for three to five minutes, bringing circulation to the area through vasodilation, which allows more blood and lymph to enter the area. A cold neck compress causing vasoconstriction and prompting constriction of the blood vessels and lymph nodes would follow. Next, the cold compress would be covered by a warm, dry towel or blanket until it dries out, which can take up to an hour. By alternating hot and cold and then allowing body heat to dry out the cold compress, congestion and stagnation are flushed from the affected area, and more immune fighting troops are brought in to heal the sore throat. This is a gentle and effective alternative to over-the-counter medications that still require a "spoonful of sugar" to help the medicine go down. Kids like this treatment, too—a game of hot and cold.

THE ENERGY WATER CONNECTION

Dr. Masaru Emoto, a researcher and author, is renowned for his groundbreaking discoveries regarding water. When exposed to harmonious music and positive human thoughts, freezing water formed beautifully designed ice crystals in Dr. Emoto's research. I suggest reading his book,

The Hidden Messages of Water, to gain a better understanding of how water is affected by our thoughts and feelings. His book is filled with excellent visuals depicting the distinctive formations of ice crystals responding to specific words, music, and physical environments. Take, as an example, repeating the words "thank you" or "hate" to water. The crystals resulting from the freezing of the "thank you" water are symmetrical and wondrous to behold. Water exposed to "hate" creates distorted and incomplete crystals.

Our bodies are 65 percent water. Hard science now reveals through brain scans, heart rate, blood pressure, and other quantitative measures that humans are certainly affected by thoughts and words. In their book, *Words Can Change Your Brain: 12 Conversation Strategies to Build Trust, Resolve Conflict, and Increase Intimacy*, neuroscientist Andrew Newberg, MD, along with Mark Robert Waldman suggest that words have the power to influence the expression of genes which regulate physical and emotional stress.[3] Perhaps in order for us to create beautifully designed lives, it's worth surrounding ourselves with positive people, positive thoughts, gratitude, and succulent real foods because these things emit "healthy vibrations." Blessed Holy Water offers hope and is believed to be sacred; so, drinking it or pure, filtered water can potentially shift one's physiology. Often, when I am enjoying a glass of water, I say "thank you" to it for offering my body energy, health, and life.

3. Andrew Newberg, MD, and Mark Robert Waldman, *Words Can Change Your Brain: 12 Conversation Strategies to Build Trust, Resolve Conflict, and Increase Intimacy*, The Penguin Group, 2012.

CHAPTER 5 HEALTH RESOLUTION

Find a beautiful, non-plastic drinking container, fill it with filtered water, and increase your daily water consumption to equal half your weight in ounces. Make a pledge to yourself, to your body, and to your health to drink half of your body weight in ounces of pure water each day. And here's a little tip: you might drink more water if you use a straw. Glass and stainless steel straws are available.

I, _____,
pledge to drink ½ my body weight in ounces of water daily. This will be my routine by this date _____ .

My weight: _____

Half my weight: _____ = the number of ounces of water I will drink each day.

Let pure, simple water work its magic and guide you to vibrancy. You may even wish to make the Hebrew toast *l'chaim*—to life—as you do so.

CHAPTER 6

Real Food

Thomas Edison once said, "The doctor of the future will give no medicine but will interest his patients in the care of the human frame, in diet, and in the cause and prevention of disease." In my way of thinking, this means that the local organic farmer could actually be the doctor of the future. If so, then I propose that "the future" is in this moment! I would rather exchange money with a local farmer today than with an oncologist tomorrow.

I WOULD RATHER EXCHANGE MONEY WITH A LOCAL FARMER TODAY THAN WITH AN ONCOLOGIST TOMORROW.

The American Diabetes Association stated in 2012 that the estimated cost of diagnosed diabetes in America was

245 billion dollars.[1] Today, in 2016, one out of every three Medicare dollars is spent managing this disease,[2] with the vast majority of money being spent on medication management, wound care, amputations, and kidney disease management. Very little is dedicated to education and disease prevention. Were we to allot even a portion of these resources to disease prevention and education of healthful life choices, we would have a thriving, robust, and creative culture. This could be accomplished if our current medical system would shift from the disease management model to one of prevention. A preventative model would include real food as the foundation to building good health. Accompanied by lifestyle education and stress management, medication would then become a last resort.

When I say "real food," I am referring to local, organic fruits and vegetables, legumes, whole grains, nuts, seeds, eggs, dairy, and meat raised without antibiotics or hormones, and open water fish. Real foods haven't been processed or refined and do not contain artificial additives. They endow our senses with bright colors, mouthwatering aromas, and deliciousness and give our entire body

1. "American Diabetes Association Releases New Research Estimating Annual Cost of Diabetes at $245 billion," American Diabetes Association, Alexandria, March 6 2013, accessed June 8, 2016, http://www.diabetes.org/newsroom/press-releases/2013/annual-costs-of-diabetes-2013.html.

2. "The Staggering Costs of Diabetes in America," American Diabetes Association, accessed June 8, 2016, http://www.diabetes.org/diabetes-basics/statistics/infographics/adv-staggering-cost-of-diabetes.html.

nourishment. Just like we want to consume clean, filtered water, we want to eat local, unadulterated, organic food.

Eating local often means eating food that is in season. Local and seasonal produce is more likely to be nutrient-dense food containing vitamins, minerals, and antioxidants, rather than preservatives, coloring, and flavor enhancers. Local produce is also more alive since it is transported fewer miles and less shocked by travel, sprays, washers, and cold storage. This week, strawberries, Minneola oranges, and dandelion greens tasted exceptionally alive to me, as they were in season in California and literally harvested from the Earth within 24 hours of my purchase and 60 miles from my home. With every bite I felt I was giving my body the gift of prolonged life.

Think about the "food" many Americans grab off shelves at gas stations and warehouse supermarkets. How fresh and "real" can a food be that has a six-month or six-year shelf life? It would be fantastic if every household in America would see the value in putting fresh seasonal strawberries purchased from a local farmer into their child's lunch box in place of dried strips of fruit pulp. Seasonal strawberries provide mouthwatering flavor, juicy texture, natural sweetness, Vitamin C, manganese, potassium, fiber, and antioxidants. Those dried up fruit roll snacks only offer a good dose of sugar, often called "concentrates," no fiber, sodium sulfate and citric acid as preservatives, added coloring to make the product look attractive, canola or other processed oils, and sometimes hidden gluten.

I'll take the juicy, June strawberry picked in the morning and placed on my tongue by the afternoon...any day!

IN SEARCH OF REAL FOOD

Real food actually does grow on trees, but most of us don't have orchards for backyards—or backyards for that matter—so where else do we find real food? I can say without hesitation that you won't find it at most traditional grocery stores or warehouses. Shop instead at a farmers market or local natural foods store, or buy from a CSA (Community Supported Agriculture). CSAs provide a week's worth of locally grown, in-season produce that is either delivered to your home or can be picked up at a certain time and location. In most parts of the country, real food ingredients plus recipes can be shipped directly to your home by innovative companies offering such services.

When all else fails, grab a grocery cart at your local health food store and stick to the perimeter. This is where you will find produce, dairy, eggs, meats, and fresh seafood—real food. When you venture into the middle of the store, the "food" offered is processed, boxed, dehydrated, bagged, frozen, and canned. Grocery conglomerates spend big bucks studying how we shop, including those of us who want to make healthy choices. Beware the aromas of baked bread and roasted chicken that make you salivate when you first walk in the door. It's precisely what the grocers want—for you to crave, feel hungry, and buy on impulse. The same is true of all those processed treats like cheddar

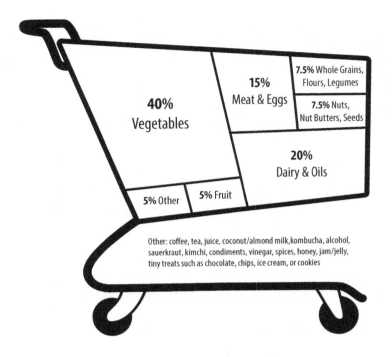

40%
Vegetables

15%
Meat & Eggs

7.5% Whole Grains,
Flours, Legumes

7.5% Nuts,
Nut Butters, Seeds

20%
Dairy & Oils

5% Other

5% Fruit

Other: coffee, tea, juice, coconut/almond milk, kombucha, alcohol,
sauerkraut, kimchi, condiments, vinegar, spices, honey, jam/jelly,
tiny treats such as chocolate, chips, ice cream, or cookies

The Health Revolution Shopping Cart

cheese croutons and caramel sauce prominently displayed in the produce aisles, and those sweet ladies handing out free tidbits. Be wary and be wise.

In most grocery stores, you enter into the produce section—mostly because it is colorful and pretty. It is also the most healthful part of the store. I suggest filling 40 percent of your cart with these luscious vegetables and fruits. Next, move to the meat counter, where you will purchase one to two pounds per person each week of fresh, antibiotic and hormone free, grass-fed meats and fish. This week I purchased two pounds of ground lamb, one pound of corned beef (for a St. Patrick's Day celebration), and one pound of chicken thighs for two of us. Of course, if you are vegetarian or vegan, you will find other forms of protein such as beans, tofu or tempeh, and quinoa. You will also want a nice selection of whole grains and legumes.

Don't forget to purchase fats such as coconut oil, olive oil, nut oils, grass-fed butter, cheese, sour cream, and cottage cheese.

Finally, reserve five percent of your cart for dark chocolate, chips, ice cream, or other indulgent delights. We all need a little treat now and then. Emphasis on *little*.

EAT A RAINBOW WITH EVERY MEAL

If you find your plate filled with "white food" and overcooked meat, as many Americans do, you are very likely not getting the nutrition you need to maintain peak health. Eating a rainbow of brightly colored foods at every meal is the way to pack in the recommended daily servings of fruits and vegetables. Colorful produce is often nutrient-dense and provides the body with substantial amounts of vitamins and minerals without adding unnecessary calories.

I grew up on Grandma's spaghetti and meatballs, maybe with some mushrooms, and a ladle of canned tomato sauce on top. The pasta provided us with carbohydrates and B12; the meatballs—protein, B2, B3, and zinc; and vitamin D came from the mushrooms. The sauce most likely had potassium, vitamins C, A, and B6, and an extremely high amount of sodium. Today, this might be considered cooking from scratch, but when it comes to nutrition and health, we can do a whole lot better.

I have learned to shake up Grandma's spaghetti with veggies, and the result is prettier, tastier, and more nutritious. (Forgive me, Grandma.) Wheat pasta would work well in this recipe (see page 82), but given that gluten is not an option in my diet, I've learned to be creative with gluten-free options.

Fruits and vegetables are loaded with phytonutrients, sometimes referred to as phytochemicals (*phyto* means plant). There are hundreds, sometimes thousands, of these chemical compounds in every bite. Different phytonutrients are responsible for the color of a fruit or vegetable, the taste, and the antioxidant properties. For example, a carrot's orange color is due to a carotenoid phytonutrient. Hundreds of carotenoids provide shades of orange, red, and yellow to our fruits and vegetables.

Phytonutrients are potent medicine. Scientists continue to study plants looking for potential drugs to market, illnesses to cure, and billions to profit. The origin of aspirin, a medicine cabinet staple, lies in the leaves and bark of the willow tree. Taxol (paclitaxel), a chemotherapy drug, is derived from Pacific Yew bark, and cardiac drugs like Digitalis come from the plant Foxglove. Plants are simply powerful!

DR. JADE'S RAINBOW SPAGHETTI FOR TWO

Spaghetti: 2 zucchini spiraled or shaved into noodles (potassium, vitamins C, A, B6, fiber). Use raw or immerse in boiling water for 30 seconds until al dente *OR* 1 spaghetti squash baked and scraped as noodles (vitamins A and B6).

Sauce: Sauté the following in a tablespoon of butter until tender-crisp.

- 1 diced yellow summer squash (vitamins A and B6)

- ½ diced yellow onion (potassium and vitamin B6)

- 2 cloves diced garlic (potassium, trace minerals such as zinc, manganese, selenium, and copper, vitamin B6)

- 2 plum tomatoes diced (antioxidants, vitamin C)

- ½ red pepper diced (antioxidants, vitamin C)

- 1 large carrot diced (antioxidants, vitamin A)

- ½ bunch of diced kale (vitamins A, C, and B6)

- 1 blue potato diced (antioxidants, fiber, potassium, and iron)

- Handful of black or Nicoise olives if desired (essential fatty acids)

Flavor with a drizzle of olive oil, chopped purple basil, any additional herbs such as oregano and thyme, sea salt, and cracked pepper or red pepper flakes for some heat. A sprinkle of dulse seaweed (iodine, trace minerals, antioxidants) makes a pretty garnish.

For added protein, dice tofu and add to the sauce.

With each new day that dawns, I invite you to enjoy at least one fruit or vegetable from every color. You could start with an egg, steamed greens, and a piece of fruit for breakfast. Enjoy green salad with shredded beets and olive oil, topped with two to three ounces of protein such as grilled organic poultry or cottage cheese for lunch. For dinner, how about steamed brown rice topped with yellow squash, tomatoes, peas, and a side of salmon followed by a small bowl of blackberries for dessert? Yum! Right?

If you have a child, ask her to play this game with you. Kids love the challenge and often bring accountability to the family.

CHOOSE YOUR MEAL'S FOOD RAINBOW

Red: beets, radishes, cabbage, Swiss chard, peppers, apples, goji berries, strawberries, raspberries, cherries, watermelon

Orange: oranges, cantaloupe, pumpkin, persimmon, sweet potatoes, apricots, butternut squash, kumquats, mangoes, papaya, nectarines, peaches, carrots, cacao, turmeric

Yellow: lemons, squash, onions, bananas, plantains, apples, grapefruit, pears, pineapple, nuts, spaghetti squash, vegetable oils, golden raisins, hemp seeds, golden flax seeds, ginger

Green: asparagus, kale, chard, spinach, dandelion greens, arugula, lettuce, avocado, celery, seaweed, string beans, peas, wheat grass, sprouts, kalettes, lime, kiwi, apples, broccoli, grapes, zucchini

Blue: blueberries, bilberries, raspberries, potatoes

Indigo: black beans, black cherries, currants, black olives, blackberries, boysenberries, plums, prunes

Violet: basil/chive flowers, purple tomatoes, dulse (seaweed), elderberries, kohlrabi, lavender, purple (red) onions, cabbage, eggplant, purple grapes, purple peppers, purple string beans, plums

Plants are vibrant and alive. They offer us a cache of energy, health, and deliciousness. Enjoy them.

MEAT & DAIRY

It is encouraging to witness younger farmers becoming involved in animal husbandry and producing locally and humanely raised organic meat. Over the past five years, red meat and poultry have become readily available at farmers markets. Now, bone broth is the hot new item due to its ability to heal the digestive tract and offer protein, fats, and overall flavor.

If you are a meat eater, look for grass-fed meat from animals raised in small lots, true free range, 100% antibiotic and hormone free, and organic if possible. Non-organic meat is loaded with antibiotics and hormones, and the animals are often fed GMO corn or other fillers. More often than not, cattle are injected with estrogen because it causes excessive water weight. (Can you relate, ladies?) Farmers are paid by the pound, and some will go to great lengths to have their cattle gain weight as quickly as possible. So, if farmer Joe can fatten his cow 25 percent by injecting hormones and feeding it GMO grains in the last few weeks before market, then farmer Joe is looking out for his pocketbook, not the health of the cow or the consumer. It is crucial to stop endorsing an industry that stuffs animals with hormones, antibiotics, and GMO grains, and crowds them into spaces with a lack of sunlight and air. This is not a humane life for any animal.

In contrast to feedlot-sourced meat, organic meat is a nutrient-dense source of real food packed with B vitamins, iron, minerals, protein, and good fats. I work diligently to encourage patients to switch to 100% organic meat (and dairy) or, at the very least, to buy from a local farmer. It's important to be aware that ground meats and sausage often include fillers such as gluten and other non-meat products. If I order sausage in a restaurant, I always ask if it is gluten-free. Most often the server does not know and will run back to the kitchen to ask. It's still a learning curve for all of us. When it comes to meat, know what you are eating.

EAT GOOD MEAT, FISH & POULTRY

Buy local, antibiotic and hormone free, organic (if possible) meat.

Beef	Lamb	Duck
Bison	Rabbit	Goose
Elk	Goat	Wild game
Venison	Chicken	Wild caught fish
Pork	Turkey	Shellfish

I recommend eating two to three ounces of meat, three to five times a week, depending upon particular health goals. It's best to look at meat as a "side dish" to the vegetables. I might have half of a sweet potato with a couple tablespoons of butter, two cups of steamed kale and spinach dressed with two tablespoons of olive oil, and three ounces of ground sirloin for dinner. And of course after dinner, it's a must to indulge in a small piece of chocolate or a small bowl of berries.

The dairy we consume should also come from pastured cows, goats, or sheep, raised free of GMO feed, antibiotics, and hormones. Pay for the best quality dairy available (raw if possible) and skip the fat-free versions. For decades we have been guided toward "fat free" foods as the healthy choice to help reduce the risk of heart disease and to stay slim. On the contrary, *natural fat in our diets does not make us fat*. In fact, it plays an essential role in heart, brain, and gut health. One example of the health benefits derived from full fat dairy is the fatty acid trans-palmitoleic acid found in milk, cheese, yogurt, and butter. It may substantially reduce the risk of type 2 diabetes (rampant in America), and it can only be obtained through diet; the body does not make it naturally.[3] A wonderful read on the relationship of different fats and obesity is *Why We Get Fat: And What to Do About It* by Gary Taubes, an award-winning science writer.

SUGGESTED DAIRY

Organic, pastured, antibiotic and hormone free, and raw if you can find it.

Cheese of all varieties	Sour cream
Cottage cheese	Whipping cream
Cream cheese	Whole milk
Half & half	Yogurt
Kefir	

GIVE THANKS

Dairy and meat products should be considered a gift of life from an animal raised with love and respect. If an animal

---

3. "Component in Common Dairy Foods May Cut Diabetes Risk," Harvard School of Public Health, hsph.harvard.edu, accessed June 6 2016, https://www.hsph.harvard.edu/news/press-releases/dairy-foods-diabetes-risk/.

is going to give its life to sustain us, let's give it the life it deserves. Let's abstain from buying animal products that are "mass" produced and instead purchase local, organic, humanely raised meat, fish, poultry, eggs, and dairy. The 2008 documentary film *Food, Inc.* may offer an incentive to stop eating fast, cheap, and unfortunately sometimes tasty meals usually made from factory farmed meat.

A DAY OF EATING

For those of you who would like some guidance, here is a sample daily menu.

Upon Waking:

- 12-16 ounces filtered water with fresh squeezed lemon or lime

Breakfast:

- 2 cups lightly steamed greens and/or vegetables, drizzled with 2-3 T olive oil and a squeeze of lemon

- 1 poached or boiled egg or 1 cup quinoa or 1 sausage

- 1 slice toast or rice cake with nut butter if you're still hungry

- 1 cup tea or coffee. If it's coffee, I go for an Americano (less caffeine than a regular cup of coffee) with 1 tsp half and half and just a hint of natural sweetener such as Stevia, honey, or maple syrup; but these additions are completely unnecessary.

Mid-morning Snack (if desired):

- ¼ cup nuts

- ½ cup fresh or frozen berries

Lunch:

- 2-3 cups steamed greens such as kale, chard, or dandelion, with ½ a sliced red pepper and a ¼ cup mushrooms. Dress with 1 T olive oil, 1 T vinegar, salt, pepper, and a few of your favorite spices.

- 2-3 ounces fish or other protein like tofu or beans

- ½ cup cooked brown rice or quinoa

- Another lunch I often enjoy is a protein-filled taco with a side salad from a local Mexican restaurant. The typical cost is under five dollars, and it includes raw vegetables (lettuce, cabbage, tomatoes, cilantro), protein (tofu or meat), salsa, fats (avocado), and carbohydrates (corn tortilla). A delicious meal and deal!

- Many of us who work find eating a nutritious lunch challenging. If you eat out, do your best to make choices that are most healthful—when in doubt use greens as a base and top it with a rainbow. If you can brown bag it, do so. Prep and pack your lunch after dinner (leftovers work well), so you can grab and go in the morning.

Afternoon Snack (if desired):

- 2 T nut butter with two celery stalks or ½ an apple and a silver dollar-sized piece of dark chocolate

- When I am feeling rather hungry, a snack I particularly like is one of the following with a kombucha to drink: an apple, orange, cup of berries, handful of nuts or seeds, or an avocado.

Dinner:

- 2-3 cups of steamed vegetables such as broccoli, cauliflower, and sweet potato drizzled with 1 T grass-fed butter

- 2-3 ounces protein (cottage cheese is a nice alternative to meat)—or you can simply double the butter or add coconut oil and have more vegetables.

- I attempt to eat my last meal of the day three hours before bedtime so my body can fully digest dinner. I don't toss and turn as much and don't have to deal with that "I'm stuffed" feeling. Sleep comes easier.

Throughout the day/between meals:

- Water. Drink half your body weight in ounces of water a day, usually separate from meals. If greatly desired, a three to four-ounce glass of water with a meal is fine. Consuming too much water with meals can prevent digestive enzymes from doing their job and may leave you feeling bloated.

FASTING

Real food is nutrition. Real food is medicine. Real food is health. Yet, digestion is a constant demand on the body, so it's considerate and wise to give it a rest. Humans have been instinctively fasting during times of illness since the beginning of humankind. We also fast for religious reasons. Preliminary research is beginning to shed light on the health benefits of fasting. Fasting (not eating for a period of time), such as the popular trend of Intermittent Fasting (IF), offers the digestive system a much-deserved vacation. It has also been shown to reduce insulin, blood sugar, triglyceride, and cholesterol levels. Those who fast report better sleep and more energy with an enhanced ability to manage stress.[4]

There are several different methods of Intermittent Fasting, but the basic idea is to split the day or week into

4. F. R. Azevedo, D. Ikeoka, B. Caramelli, "Effects of Intermittent Fasting on Metabolism in Men," Rev Assoc Med Bras (1992). 2013 Mar-Apr; 59(2):167-73, accessed June 8, 2016, http://www.ncbi.nlm.nih.gov/pubmed/23582559.

G. M. Tinsley, P. M. La Bounty, "Effects of Intermittent Fasting on Body Composition and Clinical Health Markers in Humans," www.ncbi.nih.gov, accessed June 8, 2016, Nutr Rev. 2015 Oct;73(10):661-74. doi: 10.1093/nutrit/nuv041. Epub 2015 Sep 15. Review.PMID: 26374764.

eating periods and fasting periods. An example would be to stop eating from 5:00 p.m. until lunch the next day, skipping dinner and breakfast. This provides your digestive system approximately 20 hours of blissful rest, and rewards you with more energy and insightful information as to what foods you crave. No food is allowed, but you can drink water, tea, coffee, and other non-caloric beverages.

CLEANSING DIETS

Patients often ask me about cleansing diets (also called detoxing), and which cleanse will most assuredly put their health back on track. A cleanse is a period of time, a few days to a few weeks, that you offer your body a break from the typical diet by eliminating certain foods, observing how you feel, and ideally slowing down a bit. If done properly, you will adopt some new eating habits, feel rejuvenated and, most significantly, be able to integrate what you experienced into your daily life.

Before I can provide my patients guidance with certainty, I must understand why they want to cleanse. Here are some of the "whys" I've heard over the years: "I have to lose weight." "Maybe I'll have more energy." "I want to get my mojo back." "I have a wedding to go to." "I hear it's good for you." "I've been drinking too much and need to detox." "The holidays did me in." "I want to feel better." People cleanse for all sorts of reasons, and I suggest knowing yours before starting. Having a clear intention at the outset will keep you focused. Although you can go it alone, it's often helpful and more fun to go on a cleanse with a partner. If you are new to the idea of cleansing, intend to cleanse for longer than a week, and/or have a known medical condition, seek the guidance of a licensed healthcare professional to monitor your labs and progress and to ensure the most favorable result.

There are an overwhelming number of different cleanses available to each of us. There are those that target weight loss, candida, inflammation, the liver, the colon, and the list goes on and on. One of the most revelatory cleanses I ever experienced was a sugar elimination cleanse for one month back in 2011. Perhaps it is time to do that one again, as it made a huge difference to my life. It brought to light how much sugar was hidden in the food we eat and how sugar can affect my energy level, sleep, cravings, and moods. The awareness of what sugar can do to compromise my health continues to guide me in making healthy food choices. The sugar cleanse was an early stepping-stone in my personal Health Revolution.

On the following page is a simple cleanse I recommend to patients that gives the bodily systems a rest as well as a boost of energy by cleaning out accumulated toxins. Take a break from processed foods, alcohol, caffeine, sugar—all those foods we adore, but which don't exactly nurture us. Cleansing also offers awareness of food cravings and attachments to certain foods. Many of us crave the foods that give us adverse reactions. For me, although I don't have

---

BENEFICIAL BOOSTING CLEANSE

Eliminate: alcohol, caffeine, soy, wheat, gluten, rice, oils, nuts, sugar, fruit, dairy, processed food, and all supplements except those recommended by a licensed healthcare practitioner.

Consume: 2 cups steamed and/or raw organic vegetables and one-ounce portions of wild fish or organic meat three times a day. Use apple cider vinegar and lime or lemon juice as condiments. Drink half your body weight in ounces of water daily.

---

the common symptoms of headaches and lethargy that go along with giving up coffee, I do mourn the morning ritual of brewing it, smelling it, and savoring it.

To get the most benefit, stay on my Beneficial Boosting Cleanse for at least ten days or, ideally, two weeks.

Patients notice that when they stick to the Beneficial Boosting Cleanse, they are content and feel "full" with only half the amount of food they normally eat. They also enjoy the disappearance of ailments such as headaches, joint aches, and bloating. I hope you choose to try it, especially at the start of the spring and fall seasons—a spring cleaning and a fall girding up for the holidays!

Here are some suggestions to help your cleanse be especially healing:

1. Drink half your body weight in ounces of water
    daily with fresh lemon or lime juice to stimulate
    urination and pooping in order to remove waste
    from the body.

2. Consider enemas or colonic therapy in order to fa-
    cilitate adequate bowel movements. It's important
    to assure one to two daily bowel movements while
    cleansing to obtain the maximum benefits of your
    efforts. Always engage an experienced professional
    for colonic therapy.

3. Add daily supplements (as suggested by your li-
    censed healthcare practitioner), such as liver support
    herbs, detoxification powders that assist the liver
    and the digestive system, and extra fiber or magne-
    sium if bowel movements are not happening.

4. Slow down! A cleanse is both a physical and emo-
    tional experience. Use the time dedicated to cleans-
    ing the body to also quiet the mind. This allows
    you to recognize the beneficial changes, sometimes
    quite subtle, that the cleanse brings to you. Eat and
    drink mindfully, while sitting and doing nothing
    else. Turn off and tune out all technology by 8:30
    p.m. Go to bed by ten. Walk 20 to 40 minutes dai-
    ly without your cell phone or music. Just walk to
    absorb the surroundings. Give yourself permission
    to read or journal. Essentially, take a break from
    the normal, day-to-day schedule. I have found little

to no benefit in cleansing the body if the mind and spirit are not simultaneously addressed. The movie *May I Be Frank* is a powerful portrayal of a man who uses a health cleanse as a springboard to a new life. It portrays the human ability to transform oneself. This movie, albeit an extreme situation, as the protagonist has a history of addiction and obesity, may be a catalyst for those of you wanting to create beneficial change regarding your health.

REAL FOOD DIETS

What do diets such as the *Paleo, South Beach, Slow Food, Raw Food, Mediterranean, Atkins, GAPS, FODMAP, Ketogenic, Eat Right For Your Blood Type*, and *Membrane Stabilizing*, among others, have in common? They all suggest that we eat real foods. They espouse different ratios of proteins, fats, and carbohydrates, *and* they each focus on whole foods and eschew processed food. Amen! These diets are worth experimenting with as they give you a guide—and very often delicious recipes—with which to develop what works for your body nutritionally. I have tried each of the above-mentioned diets and have learned not only about eating well, but also more about what my body does and does not like.

There are many great books and companion websites that walk you through diets step-by-step as well as provide you with mouthwatering recipes.

WHOLE FOOD BASED DIET & COOKBOOKS

The Abascal Way to Quiet Inflammation for Health and Weight Loss, Kathy Abascal

The Art of Simple Food: Notes, Lessons, and Recipes from a Delicious Revolution, Alice Waters

Crazy Sexy Kitchen: 150 Plant-Empowered Recipes to Ignite a Mouthwatering Revolution, Kris Carr and Chef Chad Sarno

Crossroads: Extraordinary Recipes from the Restaurant That Is Reinventing Vegan Cuisine, Tal Ronnen

Eat Clean Live Well, Terry Walters

Feeding the Whole Family: Recipes for Babies, Young Children, and Their Parents, Cynthia Lair

Fight Cancer with a Ketogenic Diet: A New Method for Treating Cancer, Ellen Davis

The Heal Your Gut Cookbook: Nutrient-Dense Recipes for Intestinal Health, Hilary Boynton and Mary G. Brackett

I Am Grateful: Recipes and Lifestyle of Café Gratitude, Terces Engelhart

Kitchen Matrix: More Than 700 Simple Recipes and Techniques to Mix and Match for Endless Possibilities, Mark Bittman

The Metabolic Approach to Cancer: Integrating Deep Nutrition, the Ketogenic Diet, and Nontoxic Bio-Individualized Therapies, Natasha Winters

Plenty: Vibrant Vegetable Recipes from London's Ottolenghi, Yotam Ottolenghi

Practical Paleo: A Customized Approach to Health and a Whole-Foods Lifestyle, Diane Sanfilippo and Bill Staley

The Raw Gourmet, Nomi Shannon

Super Natural Every Day: Well-Loved Recipes from My Natural Foods Kitchen, Heidi Swanson

Tacolicious: Festive Recipes for Tacos, Snacks, Cocktails, and More, Sara Deseran

Using the GAPS Diet, Hilary Boynton and Mary G. Brackett

Vegan Cooking for Carnivores: Over 125 Recipes So Tasty You Won't Miss the Meat, Roberto Martin and Quentin Bacon

Veganomicon: The Ultimate Vegan Cookbook, Isa Chandra Moskowitz and Terry Hope Romero

Vegetarian Cooking for Everyone, Deborah Madison

The Zenbelly Cookbook: An Epicurean's Guide to Paleo Cuisine, Simon Miller

The Wahls Protocol Cooking for Life: The Revolutionary Modern Paleo Plan to Treat All Chronic Autoimmune Conditions, Terry Wahls, M.D. with Eve Adamson

The more you let yourself play and experiment with diets based on real food, the more attuned you will become to the subtleties of your body. For example, I have learned that I feel much better if I eat a little protein at breakfast along with a carbohydrate like gluten-free oatmeal or a sweet potato. My energy is more abundant and my focus more directed.

FOOD AS MEDICINE

Naturopathic doctors or a good integrative physician will regularly and wholeheartedly discuss diet and lifestyle with patients. The first step in the Naturopathic Therapeutic Order is to remove obstacles to healing, and more often than not a patient's diet is a contributing factor.

Real food is a major building block to achieving health. It allows *The Vis* to flourish while minimizing the opportunity for disease to come into the picture. It's the ultimate medicine. And when I say this, I'm not referring to drinking cranberry juice for a urinary tract infection or eating bananas for leg cramps. I'm suggesting a fundamental shift in the way we, as individuals and as a culture, think of food. Food is more than calories. It has the power to lessen symptoms, nourish, and heal.

Michael Pollan offers wonderful insight in his book *In Defense of Food*. He argues food is more than micronutrients and food science, and discusses at length its role in forming relationships through sharing meals, shopping at farmers markets, and actually creating a connection with food itself by growing it. In my optimistic mind, I envision a future in which individuals and municipalities grow the majority of their own food. Local gardens will be suspended on rooftops and vertical walls, with efficient misting technology. Farming will require less water, less land, less transportation, and crops will be picked within 24 to 48 hours of going a few miles to market, thereby yielding more nutrients, fresh flavor, and vitality.

Growing, buying, and eating local, real food is at the heart of The Health Revolution. Choosing to eat organic produce, meat, and dairy from neighboring farmers producing sustenance with pride and then sharing that sustenance with those we love is a win-win for all. Consuming real food can be one of the most ethical things we do for ourselves, our planet, and all living things.

———————

CHAPTER 6 HEALTH RESOLUTIONS

1. I will commit to shopping once a week at a farmers market for one entire month.

2. I will invite friends to my house or a local park and share food, love, and laughter.

3. I will put this note on my fridge:

> EAT REAL FOOD.
> EAT REAL FOOD.
> EAT REAL FOOD.

To help you commit to the above, sign here:

_____

4. For a quick and entertaining education on all the reasons why what we eat is so very crucial, I will watch a movie such as *Super Size Me*, *GMO OMG*, *Food, Inc.*, *Forks Over Knives*, or *Fed Up*. Each film offers viewpoints and facts worth contemplating.

CHAPTER 7
———

Supplements:
The 21 Billion Dollar Industry

Americans are not shy about filling their shopping carts with supplements—literally tons of them. According to *Healthline*, an online news source, Americans were projected to spend a whopping 21 billion dollars on supplements in 2015.[1] That's about ten times more than what Americans spent on legal cannabis in 2014, which was 2.7 billion dollars according to market research from ArcView Group, a cannabis investment and research firm.[2] Looking at sales of supplements and cannabis alone suggests that many

1. Cameron Scott, "Americans Spend Billions on Vitamins and Herbs That Don't Work," *Healthline*, March 19, 2015, accessed February 11, 2016, http://www.healthline.com/health-news/americans -spend-billions-on-vitamins-and-herbs-that-dont-work-031915.
2. Matt Ferner, "Legal Marijuana is the Fastest-Growing Industry in the U.S.: Report," *Huffington Post*, January 28, 2015, accessed February 12, 2016, http://www.huffingtonpost.com/2015/01/26/marijuana-industry-fast-est-growing_n_6540166.html.

Americans are searching outside of insurance plans and the traditional Western medical paradigm to receive the help they need.

The question begging to be answered is: "What are we trying to assist or fix?" All too often, we rely on supplements as the magical elixir. We want them to treat, prevent, and enhance our lives. These desires make it easy to market supplements. They sound tantalizing because we want a pill or cream to cure us of some undesirable state. I see it differently. Our bodies have the ability to balance themselves when they are running in optimal form. Supplements should be used judiciously to assist bodily systems. Per the Naturopathic Therapeutic Order, lifestyle and stabilization of bodily systems should be addressed first when working with a patient, and supplementation can often expedite the stabilizing.

I am not in favor of taking an over-abundance of supplements, though at times they play a significant role in offsetting our individual health handicaps, or barriers, to proper diet and nutrition. Since much of our food is grown in depleted soil and then processed, many of us benefit from supplementation. According to a study published in 2004 by the University of Texas, over the past 50 years, 43 different fruits and vegetables had declines in protein, calcium, phosphorous, iron, vitamin B2, and vitamin C. These declines were due to agricultural practices that focused on improving size, pest resistance, and growth rate of food—not nutrition.[3]

Supplements can help furnish the vitamins, minerals, amino acids, enzymes, and antioxidants that our foods now lack. This is the "good stuff" that supports the body and mind—allowing us to perform at our peak. Today's American diet is often deficient in nutrients such as omega-3 essential fatty acids (EFAs). EFAs are known to enhance cognitive function, improve cardio-vascular function, and decrease general inflammation throughout the body. If you are vegan or vegetarian, for example, it would behoove you to consume an omega-3 supplement because often you don't obtain enough EFAs from plants. If you have iron deficient anemia, it's wise to first figure out the root cause, and then supplement while you address the why. And many of us do not get enough sun, so taking vitamin D is beneficial when our levels are below optimal. These are legitimate and healing ways to use supplements.

A CASE STUDY

Not too long ago, a fifty-year-old woman came to me with an acute sinus infection. She had been dealing with three to four such infections a year for some time and was tired of taking antibiotics. I immediately told her I would help treat

3. "Dirt Poor: Have Fruits and Vegetables Become Less Nutritious?" Scientific American, EarthTalk®, April 27, 2011, accessed January 31, 2016, http://www.scientificamerican.com/article/soil-depletion-and-nutrition-loss.

the current infection, but just as importantly, we would work together to prevent them in the future.

The wellness plan I suggested included vitamin C, zinc, vitamin D, and a botanical tincture of antimicrobial herbs to build her immune system and help mitigate the infection. I also recommended the daily use of a neti pot to flush out her sinuses. Flushing the nasal passages with treated water from a neti pot is an Ayurvedic practice. A neti pot resembles a small teapot and may be purchased in most health food stores or drugstores. I advised her to eliminate dairy from her diet for four weeks. For many, dairy is mucous forming, and you don't need more of that when you are dealing with a sinus infection. I also counseled her to hydrate with water and increase her intake immensely. She began the wellness plan, and within a week she felt significantly better without the use of antibiotics.

Her treatment, however, didn't stop there. We created a three-month plus prevention plan, in which supplementation was integral. I recommended three grams of vitamin C and 25 mg of zinc taken twice a day, and two probiotic capsules daily. These products supported her while she did the major work of changing her lifestyle. This included purchasing new hypoallergenic pillows; decreasing dairy intake to organic half-and-half with her morning coffee; cutting back on sugars like candy and milk chocolate; consuming more nourishing foods like bone broth, berries, and protein doused with turmeric and ginger; and considering a huge change: giving up smoking cigarettes. In my clinical experience, smokers tend to have a higher incidence of sinus infections so addressing this habit is crucial. Smoking is a very difficult habit to quit, and yet, patients who have a strong commitment and solid support can achieve this goal.

It's my job to nudge clients in the direction of health. Supplements prescribed to assist in lifestyle change and address underlying reasons for disease are effective and ethical. If I had only given this patient a supplement to kill the infection, and not addressed any lifestyle behaviors, I would be joining the status quo of healthcare. Suggesting a supplement without addressing the underlying issue is known as "green allopathy." Alternative healthcare professionals can do better than that.

IT'S MY JOB TO NUDGE CLIENTS IN THE DIRECTION OF HEALTH.

Before an ad on your social media page or a product endorsed by a favorite celebrity seduces you, I suggest working with your chosen healthcare practitioner. Team up with someone who reinforces your health goals and implements appropriate supplements as a part of your total wellness plan—someone who works diligently to keep cost and number of pills swallowed to a minimum.

HOW MANY SUPPLEMENTS ARE TOO MANY?

I have a friend who organizes people's homes, and she says it is very common for her to find kitchen cupboards full of unused, outdated supplements worth hundreds, if not thousands, of dollars.

I try to keep the number of supplements a patient is taking to a minimum, clarifying specifically why each is needed. Additionally, our bodies are cyclical, just like the seasons; therefore, the supplements we consume should also change. It's winter as I write this, so I am taking a few products to help maintain my health: liquid fish oil to promote cognitive functioning and skin health, a probiotic for immune and digestive support, an additional immune system support, vitamin D3/K2 due to the lack of sunshine on my skin, and a blended mushroom formula that offers stamina and additional immunity. That's a total of five. I have been traveling extensively, and blood tests show that my cortisol levels bounce up and down with the lack of sleep, the added stress, and the increased consumption of unfamiliar foods and restaurant food that accompany travel. Supporting my adrenal glands (where cortisol is made) with supplements helps stabilize my blood sugar and sleep, and keeps me chugging along (not buzzing, as with caffeine) through the long, bustling days and all-too-short nights. Currently, my adrenal support is a Siberian ginseng solid extract mixed with a hawthorn berry solid extract.

The take home regarding supplementation is this: a supplement should be used to assist the body in accomplishing what it can't do on its own and for a finite window of time. For instance, it might be in your best interest to take Coenzyme Q10 (CoQ10) if you are on a cholesterol lowering medication, since it's indisputable that this enzyme is often depleted by the medication. CoQ10 provides cells with energy and protects against cardio-vascular damage; for that reason, supplementing while you and your doctor figure out why your body is producing extra cholesterol is wise. Chances are, with diet and lifestyle changes, over time both the medication and CoQ10 will no longer be needed.

SUPPLEMENT FORM

Eighty percent of supplements taken by my patients are in oral form, whether that is a pill, capsule, liquid, or chewable. Some supplements are also available as suppositories, intramuscular injections, patches, creams, ointments, and IVs.

When purchasing supplements, do so from a trusted source and not a drugstore or grocery store. Licensed healthcare professionals and reputable supplement companies invest ample amounts of time, research, and money to attend conferences where they learn about the latest research and clinical applications of products. Most naturopathic and integrated doctors sell products directly to patients as a way of convenience. Most importantly, they have the clinical experience to know what works and what is safe. That doesn't mean you shouldn't investigate and learn for yourself. It's easy to utilize Pubmed.com and other online resources to learn up-to-the-minute research and data on a particular product.

DR. JADE'S SUPPLEMENT RECOMMENDATIONS

Supplementation is just one of my eight guidelines for living a wonderful life. Eating real food and drinking water, developing community, de-stressing, and moving the body aren't effectively replaced by a capsule. And yet, the right supplement(s) can be a strong building block when shoring up a body that is out of balance.

Here are a few supplements I commonly recommend. Please do not run out and purchase all of these and begin taking them at random. Work with a licensed healthcare professional to address your unique health goals and make sure the supplements chosen are the ones your body needs. You will notice that many of the supplements recommended vary with the seasons. Our bodies are part of nature and constantly changing. I recognize the need to shift supplementation with the ebb and flow of the year. I invite you to do the same.

YEAR ROUND AND SEASONAL SUPPLEMENT SUGGESTIONS
Dr. Jade Wimberley, ND

Year Round		
Supplement	*Possible Benefit*	*Dosage*
Methyl B Complex	Increases energy and mental clarity	1-2 capsules QD* or BID** with food
Magnesium Glycinate or Citrate	Increases energy, helps stabilize blood sugar, promotes consistent bowel movements	1 capsule QD or BID
Digestive Enzymes	Enhances nutrient absorption with less bloating, gas, and discomfort	PRN*** with meals or larger snacks
Adrenal Support	Increases energy, promotes sound sleep, thyroid support	1-2 teaspoons or capsules QD or BID
Medicinal Mushrooms	Enhances the immune system: sick less with more stamina	1-2 capsules QD or BID
Spring		
Probiotics	Provides immune and digestive support, less bloating and gas. Often helps with mental health conditions.	1-2 capsules BID

Supplement	Possible Benefit	Dosage
Liver Support	Increases energy and detoxification, supports the skin	1-2 capsules BID
Liquid Fish Oil	Supports bowel and skin health, cognitive enhancement	1-2 grams BID
Summer		
R Lipoic Acid	An antioxidant, stabilizes blood sugar	200 mg QD or BID
Zinc	An antioxidant and antiviral, enhances male fertility	25-50 mg QD or BID
Melatonin	An antioxidant, promotes sound sleep	1-2 mg HS****
Vitamin C	Antioxidant and antiviral	1-5 grams BID
Fall		
Immune System Support	Enhances the immune system: sick less with more stamina	1-2 caps QD or BID
Vitamin D3/ K2	Supports the immune system and bone health	1,000-5,000 IUs /45 mcg QD
Liquid Fish Oil	Supports bowel and skin health, cognitive enhancement	1-2 grams BID

Supplement	Possible Benefit	Dosage
Winter		
Liquid Fish Oil	Supports bowel and skin health, cognitive enhancement	1-2 grams BID
Probiotics	Provides immune and digestive support, less bloating and gas. Often helps with mental health conditions.	1-2 capsules BID
Vitamin D3/ K2	Supports the immune system and bone health	1,000-5,000 IUs /45 mcg QD
Immune System Support	Enhances the immune system: sick less with more stamina	1-2 caps QD or BID

*QD = daily   **BID = twice daily
***PRN = as needed   ****HS = at bedtime

SUPPLEMENTS TO CONSIDER YEAR ROUND

I rarely suggest that a particular supplement be taken all of the time. Yet, there are a few from which most of my patients benefit regularly. The top five that I feel give the most bang for your buck when it comes to augmenting overall stamina and disease prevention are: Methyl-B Complex, magnesium glycinate or citrate, digestive enzymes, an adrenal support, and medicinal mushrooms. Let's take a brief look at each.

Methyl-B Complex: This supplement contains all the B vitamins and choline and inositol. Methyl-B complex augments energy production, immunity, cardiovascular health, anemia, and many neurological imbalances. It aids in helping us manage our hectic lifestyles.

Magnesium Glycinate or Citrate: All forms of magnesium are not created equal, so be knowledgeable about the form you are taking and why. I most often prescribe magnesium glycinate if I suspect someone is magnesium deficient, and magnesium citrate if the patient tends to have constipation. Magnesium is a go-to for all sorts of conditions including but not limited to insomnia, fatigue, headaches, constipation, and body aches and pains.

Digestive Enzymes: This supplement is often needed to encourage digestion of meals as well as larger snacks. The enzymes help break down your food more efficiently so your body can use the nutrients for energy and building blocks. I often suggest using enzymes when eating at restaurants or traveling. There are many versions: those with or without hydrochloric acid, botanical tinctures, pancreatic enzymes, and some even contain ox bile. Once again, it's important to work with a professional to help you discern which enzyme is best suited to your digestive needs.

Adrenal Support: Thyroid function, or more accurately dysfunction, garners the most attention from mainstream medicine, while the adrenal glands are too often neglected. Integrative healthcare providers know how to test for adrenal fatigue and how to support the adrenals with supplementation. This can help alleviate exhaustion and reduce stress by regulating the hormone cortisol. There are many adrenal support products available, each with different merit and properties. Some of my favorites are Siberian ginseng, particular B vitamins, licorice root, Holy Basil, DHEA, and adrenal blends. Consuming stimulants, alcohol, sugar, and simple carbohydrates may exacerbate adrenal fatigue, so lifestyle and diet should be addressed in conjunction with supplementation.

Medicinal Mushroom Blend: Mushrooms are actually a whole food and not an isolated vitamin or mineral such as vitamin C or magnesium, respectively. Mushrooms contain a plethora of nutrients that work synergistically to boost the immune, cardiovascular, and respiratory systems. I see vast improvement in patients who have depleted immune systems (aka get sick a lot) with the help of mushroom supplements. Mushroom blends also promote a healthy gut. Mushroom research is expanding in regards to the many health benefits and potential uses of these edible fungi. Paul Stamets, author, speaker and mycologist, is a leader in the "mushrooms as medicine" movement. He's one to have on your radar, and you can begin by checking out his TED talk.

CHANGING WITH THE SEASONS

Spring is the time to cleanse and build up your body as you come out of winter's hibernation. There is now more sunlight and life gears up, just like the seeds in the garden sprout and root.

SPRING SUPPLEMENTS

Probiotics: A great variety of these helpful microorganisms are stocked on health food store, grocery store, and pharmacy shelves across the country. Probiotics are live bacteria that benefit our health in multiple ways. Supplements will often be categorized by the strain(s) and volume of bacteria offered, each with a specific benefit to digestion, the immune system, vaginal health, and the sinuses. Probiotics also rebalance bodily systems after a course, or courses, of antibiotics, and they increase vitamin B12 absorption. Vitamin B12 plays vital roles in human health by maintaining nerve and blood cells and in making DNA. The Human Food Project, a non-profit organization, collects, researches, and shares information on the role of probiotics in the human body. You can investigate this group and their mission further by visiting Humanfoodproject.com.

Probiotics, consisting of live bacteria and yeast, can be obtained from fermented foods such as sauerkraut, kefir, yogurt, miso, kombucha, tempeh, and kimchi. And yet, supplementation is often justified, especially when a patient has been on antibiotics or has digestive distress. I often begin patients on a starter kit of lactobacillus and bifidobacterium, two of the most commonly known probiotics, and adjust from there.

Probiotics are indicated:

- after a course of antibiotics to restore healthy intestinal or vaginal flora,

- to maintain a healthy gut, especially while traveling abroad,

- when fending off a cold,

- before and after a dental cleaning, and

- for numerous digestive issues.

I also consider them as an auxiliary treatment for depression, anxiety, and chronic fatigue. The gut is our second brain, and a happy gut often means a happy brain. Probiotics are also beneficial in the winter because we tend to eat fewer whole foods and more processed foods and sugar over the holidays.

Liver Support: Think of the liver as the body's oil filter, except it's filtering all your blood. (You probably pay more attention to oil changes than your liver health, don't you?) A liver support supplement aids in the daily elimination of toxins and in the management of inflammatory responses throughout the body. There are many varieties of liver support products to choose from including milk thistle, peppermint, turmeric, dandelion root, and glutathione. I strongly encourage you to discuss this topic with your licensed healthcare professional to find the formula that will service you best.

Liquid Fish Oil: I prescribe this supplement in the spring because patients are cleansing and fish oil is excellent for promoting bowel movements. More on this supplement coming up in the Fall Supplement section.

Summer is the time to venture outdoors and to celebrate with those you love, drinking in those long sunshiny days, and perhaps, a libation or two. Nurture and protect your body, so you can bloom to your full potential.

SUMMER SUPPLEMENTS

R-Lipoic Acid: This powerful antioxidant helps repair the damage to cells that free radicals can cause. In the summer, free radicals come in the form of lots of sun and increased alcohol consumption. There's also the go-go-go factor to consider while we vacation and enjoy outdoor activities. R-lipoic acid helps the body turn sugar into energy. R-lipoic acid is also quite effective in protecting the liver and in regulating blood sugar. I recommend it to patients who are pre-diabetic, diabetic, and who consume more than one alcoholic drink a night. (This sometimes happens on hot summer weekends.)

Zinc: Zinc is an immune modulator, which is often deficient in people who become sick regularly, and especially those dealing with viruses. If this is true for you, it's a good supplement to consider within a comprehensive wellness plan. It's often recommended to men to help increase their sperm mobility and count, consequently increasing fertility. Zinc is also known to lower levels of copper. Elevated levels of copper have been linked to poor immunity, attention deficit disorder, acne, depression, and other undesirable conditions.

Melatonin: Melatonin is both a potent antioxidant and an essential building block for the "happiness inducing" molecule, serotonin. For most, sleep and happiness go hand in hand. I often suggest herbs as a sleep aid; however, when a patient is struggling specifically with falling into a healthy sleep pattern, melatonin is useful. I find myself recommending melatonin mostly in the summer, because that's when the majority of us experience the most struggle with sleep. The sun is out much longer, and it's harder to settle into a good night's rest.

Vitamin C (ascorbic acid): The most underrated antioxidant on the market is vitamin C. Vitamin C is a proven antiviral, immune booster, and overall antioxidant for your body. Take plain old, inexpensive ascorbic acid if your stomach will allow, and if not, look for a formula buffered by a bioflavonoid (a yellow, plant-based buffer).

Fall is the time to listen to and sustain your body. Just like the leaves change from green to orange, gold, and burgundy, your body shifts into a time of reflection and needs protection.

FALL SUPPLEMENTS

Immune System Support: Fall is a great time to start boosting the immune system in preparation for the colds and flus that are sure to be circulating throughout the winter. There are many immune support supplements to choose from, and most of my patients benefit from medicinal mushrooms. Nonetheless, there are other immunity boosters to consider. Some of my favorites are Oregon grape root, burdock, astragalus, and Echinacea. And please, don't forget the healing powers of real food. Stew and soup season is on!

Vitamin D3 with K2: The latest research backs up taking vitamin D3 and K2 together to increase cardiovascular and bone health while supporting the immune system. The dosage depends upon your current levels determined by blood tests. Because the fall and winter days are shorter, most patients benefit from vitamin D3 with K2 during both seasons.

Liquid Fish Oil: I recommend liquid fish oil made of sardines and anchovies. With liquid you obtain more anti-inflammatory omega-3 oil per teaspoon than with a handful of large capsules. Fish oil aids cognitive function, decreases inflammatory processes, contributes to cardiovascular health, regulates bowel movements, and enhances skin health. I usually prescribe liquid fish oil during the fall and winter to provide insulation during cold weather. It helps prevent dry, cracked skin, and healthy skin is a barrier to flus and colds.

Winter is the time to slow down, hibernate, and store energy. It's the most common time for flus, colds, and coughs, so protect yourself with nourishing broths and soups. Incorporate spices such as ginger, clove, pepper, cardamom, and garlic into your cooking. Do like those big, burly bears and take the time to sleep, as the outside is blanketed in snow.

WINTER SUPPLEMENTS

During the winter, I recommend liquid fish oil, probiotics, vitamin D3/K2, and immune system support supplements, all of which have been addressed in the earlier seasons.

ADDITIONAL FORMS OF SUPPLEMENTATION

In addition to vitamins, minerals, amino acids, and other supplements found in capsule form, I use botanical tinctures (liquid medicine made from whole plants) and teas. I enjoy blending tinctures and teas as indicated by my patients' health goals.

Some of the beautiful herbs I use in tinctures are passionflower, hawthorn, licorice, Vitex, elderberry, chamomile, green tea, milk thistle, Siberian ginseng, nettles, ginger, turmeric, garlic, dandelion root and leaf, lemon balm, prickly pear, osha root, Echinacea, Oregon grape root, Holy Basil, and calendula.

Tinctures are powerful medicine as they are liquid and readily absorbed by the body. They do not have to be digested or broken down like a food, capsule, or tablet. If a tincture is held in the mouth for 10 to 20 seconds, the medicine will absorb into the circulatory system sublingually, and the effects can be felt immediately. Dosage depends on the tincture blend, the health goal, and the individual's health, but it usually ranges from a few drops to a few droppers full every day.

A revered mentor of mine, the late Dr. Bill Mitchell, ND, said, "You can like tinctures all day long, but if your patient isn't going to take them, then they're not going to work." This is true. Since we have become a capsule culture, I often have to encourage patients to try a tincture. Most people are unfamiliar with tinctures or had a bad childhood experience with liquid medicine. When I can convince a patient to try this form of supplementation, it has been very successful. Tinctures often become preferred over capsules.

NUTRITIONAL IVS

There is one more supplement I find invaluable as it helps maintain overall wellness and assists in recovery from conditions ranging from dehydration to cancer. I prescribe it regularly in my practice: the nutritional IV.

Nutritional IVs are garnering a great deal of press these days as a hangover cure and the medicine of choice for celebrities. However, they have uses that are much more profound and beneficial than this.

I offer nutritional IVs to most of my patients dealing with acute situations such as flu, infection (chronic and acute), dehydration, migraines, fatigue, PMS, anxiety, depression, insomnia, peripheral neuropathy (damage to the peripheral nervous system), cancer, and chronic pain.

An IV can be administered after a catheter is inserted into a vein, most often in the arm, allowing the solution to drip into the blood stream. The patient may work, read, or rest during the 15-minute to three-hour treatment. Unlike oral supplements, the nutrients in an IV do not have to go through digestion; they go directly into the blood stream for immediate use. In 95 percent of acute situations, patients recover more rapidly when they are given nutritional IVs that provide vitamins, minerals, amino acids, and other substances that bolster health.

I find nutritional IVs indispensable to patients diagnosed with cancer. They help sustain the patient undergoing chemotherapy or radiation by supporting the immune system, thereby reducing the risk of secondary infection, preventing nerve damage, and hydrating the body. This can help a patient avoid hospitalization due to a secondary infection, which can literally save his or her life.

If you and your doctor feel nutritional IV therapy could be beneficial, choose a practiced, licensed healthcare professional who will offer you peace of mind, especially if you are new to nutritional IVs.

SUPPLEMENT SUMMARY

Supplements are part of an integrated doctor's toolbox for healing, and yet, I stress that supplementation should not and does not trump the importance of eating real food, de-stressing, moving, and soaking up community support. Supplements benefit health while you revitalize weak spots with a foundational wellness plan. Pay attention to your body, identify where it needs help, and work with your licensed healthcare practitioner to take the guessing game out of gaining and maintaining ideal health. The more you understand your body and are able to bolster weak links with the occasional supplement, the more power and energy you'll have.

CHAPTER 7 HEALTH RESOLUTIONS

1. Remove all supplements (and prescriptions if applicable) from your cabinets, refrigerator, medicine chest, closets, drawers, and nightstands. Properly dispose of anything that is expired, or that you simply never use. Place the remainder in a bag and rejoice that you have taken the first step in creating

a wellness plan. To help you commit to this, sign here when step one is complete:

_____

2. Make an appointment with a licensed healthcare professional who will take the time necessary to discuss your health goals. Take your bag of remaining goodies to your chosen professional, and decide which products stay and which ones go. I have done this with hundreds of patients; so, don't be shy, as we doctors have seen it all. Empower yourself by continuing to take only those supplements that are beneficial to your health. Have you completed this step? Awesome, then sign away:

_____

3. Use these steps as a springboard to developing a focused and beneficial wellness plan that is unique to you and your body.

CHAPTER 8

Harmonious Hormones

When you hear the word "hormone," what comes to mind? Got it? Good. What came up for you? Over the past year, I've asked friends, colleagues, and patients this same question and received answers such as: "powerful," "wild," "my wife," "emotional," "unpredictable," "PMS," "sex drive," "no sex drive," "youth," and "tears." Was your answer similar?

Responses such as these would make a fabulous YouTube video titled *What Are These Folks Talking About?* Hormones are fascinating, incredible, and sometimes troublemakers. It's interesting and not necessarily surprising that the word "hormone" has become linked to the idea that something is off-kilter or has gone a little bit "crazy." Trial lawyers even argue that clients were under the influence of their off-kilter hormones when they committed homicide or other malicious crimes. There is some truth behind the idea of "raging" hormones, and, accordingly, the idea of soothing or balancing them makes sense.

The word "hormone" comes from a Greek root meaning "that which sets in motion." This is because hormones are chemical messengers that create change in our bodies. Hormones play a role in mood, sleep, energy, pleasure, weight, sexuality, fertility, hair growth, skin health, and so much more. They're vital to health from the beginning of life. It takes a sperm and an egg to make an embryo, and what aids in that miracle happening? Hormones. Estrogen, thyroid stimulating hormone, testosterone, insulin, and progesterone are integral to this age-old miracle.

Throughout your entire life, the maintenance of desirable hormone levels will keep you vital, more balanced, and energized. Harmonious hormones can be integral to optimum health. That's why balancing patient hormones is one of the guidelines of my practice.

The act of balancing hormones is both an art and a science. The *art* is listening to patients' concerns and prescribing hormones for each patient's exact needs. Not only must the doctor listen, the patient must learn to pay attention to his or her body so as to provide accurate information to the doctor. The *science* provides the objective data—the physical exam, analyzing lab test results, and determining the level and type of hormone replacement necessary.

> THE ACT OF BALANCING HORMONES IS BOTH AN ART AND A SCIENCE.

It's too bad a "check engine" light doesn't glow on your dashboard telling you to balance your hormones. Thankfully, though, I do see medical technology heading in this direction. One medical device that collects objective data is the diabetic insulin pump. It determines glucose levels and then pumps insulin (a hormone) into the body to maintain a functional level. The pump eliminates the need for diabetics to manually check their blood sugars. Though the pump still has its imperfections, it's one example of how practical hormone monitoring and technology have advanced together.

THE ENDOCRINE SYSTEM

Glands located throughout the body produce hormones that are then distributed to other glands, organs, tissues, and cells, stimulating each to do their job and keeping our bodies functioning. Collectively, these glands are known as the endocrine system.

At this moment, while you're reading, the glands of your endocrine system are secreting 40 different hormones. Hormones play a significant role in such sensations as hunger, body temperature, mood, sleepiness, and sex drive. Exactly how all these hormones are produced is a complicated conversation. Suffice it to say, for now, that hormone production includes genetics, protein synthesis, and the work of cholesterol building blocks. Cholesterol is not all bad, as some medical reports have made out in the past. It plays a crucial role in producing many of our sex hormones,

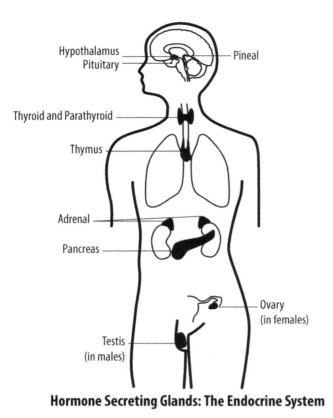

Hypothalamus
Pituitary
Pineal
Thyroid and Parathyroid
Thymus
Adrenal
Pancreas
Ovary
(in females)
Testis
(in males)

Hormone Secreting Glands: The Endocrine System

such as cortisol, estrogen, testosterone, progesterone, and DHEA (dehydroepiandrosterone). The exact workings of the endocrine system are somewhat mystifying and a bit of a marvel.

The modern day lifestyle, comprised of relentless schedules, processed food, and a polluted environment, wreaks havoc on the endocrine system, which regulates the activity of cells and/or organs—a huge and multi-faceted job. That's why balancing hormones often becomes, and rightfully so, an integral part of a comprehensive wellness plan.

THE HPA AXIS

Balancing the HPA axis is all the buzz these days in the medical world. Google it, and you will find a plethora of links pairing the HPA axis with words like stress, adrenal fatigue, depression, dysfunction, suppression, and functional medicine. You seemingly have to fix it, regulate it, and reset it. So, what is it and why is it so important?

The HPA axis is the main circuit of the body's hormonal system that includes the hypothalamus (H) and pituitary (P) glands in the brain and the adrenal glands (A) sitting right above each kidney. Hence, these three different glands are called the HPA axis. It's called an "axis" because these glands are the main line of communication for our fight or flight response.

The hypothalamus and pituitary glands are the conductors of the body's hormonal "symphony" and receive "action item" messages from the adrenal glands as well as other glands throughout the body. All of these glands work together, constantly monitoring and controlling sensations and processes ranging from blood sugar levels, sleep patterns, hunger, body temperature, energy levels, and stress response. Metabolism and immune and inflammatory responses are also part of the hormonal functions conducted by the HPA axis.

Related to the HPA axis and its myriad responsibilities is adrenal fatigue. The adrenal glands are principal players in fine-tuning the entire endocrine system. When the adrenals are in tune, your hormones (and hence you) ebb and flow like a symphony instead of a middle school band practice. When the adrenal glands create high cortisol levels that fluctuate every day, year after year (often coinciding with blood sugar levels), adrenal fatigue is the result. Excessive sluggishness, weight changes, moodiness, and sleep issues are all symptoms of such a hormonal imbalance, and adrenal support is often warranted. It's essential to partner with a doctor who understands how to address adrenal fatigue. Mainstream medicine often addresses only thyroid and blood sugar levels with medications such as levothyroxine and metformin. As an alternative, there are numerous lifestyle changes, supplements, and herbs that can return adrenal functioning to a normal level. Medication may never be necessary.

THYROID AND RELATED HORMONES

One out of three women today has a thyroid condition. If it is detected, the patient is most often prescribed levothyroxine, the second most commonly prescribed drug in America, with about 28.3 million prescriptions filled yearly.[1] Though men can develop thyroid disease and thyroid cancer, it's much more common for women. The jury is still out as to why so many women are diagnosed with thyroid disease. This might be explained by the tendency for

1. "WHO Model List of Essential Medicines" 18th list, April 2013, Amendments October 2013, accessed September 18, 2015, http://www.who. int/medicines/publications/essentialmedicines/en/.

women to have more autoimmune diseases in general than men, or because women go to the doctor more often than men and, as a result, are diagnosed.

It is very possible for a person to have a thyroid condition and for it to go undetected. This is the reason that thyroid labs should be run annually. I investigate the possibility of a thyroid condition with many of my new patients, male and female, as this can often be what's contributing to the common complaints of fatigue, weight gain, variations in temperature, and emotional upset. In addition, the symptoms of thyroid imbalances can mimic mental health conditions such as depression, ADD, and anxiety. Before a patient turns to medication for these, I suggest all thyroid levels be determined. Also, if a patient has seen little success from thyroid treatment, including medication, this prompts me to ask the patient if she has had her thyroid antibodies checked. If antibodies are present, the thyroid should be supported, but support for the adrenal glands and the immune system is also warranted. Antibodies attack and may destroy the thyroid over time, so it is prudent to keep them in check.

THE SYMPTOMS OF THYROID IMBALANCES CAN MIMIC MENTAL HEALTH CONDITIONS SUCH AS DEPRESSION, ADD, AND ANXIETY.

Thyroid dysfunction is a multi-layered medical condition and just taking a prescription is often a band-aid approach. Extensive lab analysis and changes in diet and lifestyle can result in management that does not include taking thyroid medication or removing the thyroid. If a patient has been put on a thyroid prescription or supplement, labs should be monitored every three to six months at first and then every six to 12 months after that to determine treatment efficacy. In many cases, medication can be discontinued once the underlying cause of the condition is addressed. However, if the thyroid has been removed or ablated, discontinuing thyroid medication is not an option.

During a physical examination of the thyroid, the doctor palpates the throat and asks the patient to swallow. This is to detect goiters, masses, or any other irregularities of the thyroid gland. It takes blood tests, though, to learn exactly what is happening with the thyroid hormones. If functioning efficiently, the process occurs like this: thyroid

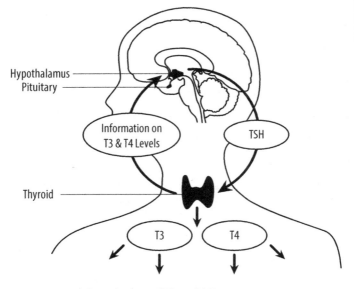

Regulation of Thyroid Hormones

stimulating hormone (TSH) from the pituitary gland signals the thyroid to produce or not to produce two thyroid hormones. These are T3 and T4, which vary due to the number of iodine molecules each holds (three or four). T3 and T4 are then released into the blood stream and travel throughout the body, controlling metabolism, heart and digestive functions, muscles, brain development, and the prevention of osteoporosis. The thyroid feeds back information to the brain regarding how much T4 and T3 is being produced. Variances in TSH, T4, and T3 levels determine if a patient is diagnosed with normal thyroid function, hypothyroidism, hyperthyroidism, or thyroid cancer.

TYPES OF THYROID DISEASE

Hypothyroidism occurs when the thyroid is underactive and fails to produce a sufficient amount of the T4 and T3 hormones. This can be confusing because in hypothyroidism the TSH level is actually elevated. Patients often feel cold and experience weight gain, hair loss, constipation, lack of sex drive, and general fatigue if they have an underactive thyroid. Hypothyroidism can also mimic depression, so it's essential to have

HYPOTHYROIDISM CAN ALSO MIMIC DEPRESSION.

your labs checked yearly to determine if the low you are feeling is due to hypothyroidism.

Hyperthyroidism—the opposite of hypothyroidism—occurs with overproduction of thyroid hormones. Consequently, in this condition, TSH will be low and at times very close to a 0.00 value. This translates into patients who have lots of energy, unexplained weight loss, insomnia, and diarrhea. It can mimic ADHD, anxiety, mania, and bipolar disorder. Many people will live in a state of hyperthyroidism for quite some time, thinking they are dealing with other disorders, but if this goes unchecked, more serious medical issues can arise such as heart attack and stroke. Often, a person with Hashimoto's autoimmune disease will experience a period of hyperthyroidism for months, up to a year, then the hyper state fades into hypothyroidism. This is when most people run to their doctors. No one likes hypothyroid symptoms, though many will live with hyperthyroid symptoms for some time.

Hashimoto's autoimmune disease occurs when the immune system attacks the thyroid. It causes chronic inflammation and, as a consequence, the thyroid gland may fail completely over time. Many people diagnosed with hypothyroidism have never been tested for Hashimoto's. It's critical to know whether or not your thyroid condition is autoimmune so you can be monitored and treated accordingly. Symptoms may include weight gain, fatigue, constipation, feeling cold, joint and muscle pain, hair loss, irregular periods, and difficulty becoming pregnant.

Overall, thyroid health is a big-time player in everyday metabolism, influencing energy level, focus, body temperature, our ability to lose or gain weight, and even our daily pooping schedule! Ask your doctor to order thyroid labs, or at bare minimum the TSH level, as part of your annual checkup. And certainly, partner with an integrative doctor who can recommend different lifestyle choices, diet enhancements, and perhaps a few supplements to benefit your overall thyroid health.

SEX HORMONES

All hormone levels fluctuate throughout our lives, and sex hormones are no exception. A teen-aged boy, a pregnant woman, a menopausal woman, a man in "middle-age crisis," and a woman with PMS or polycystic ovary syndrome are all well known examples of sex hormone fluctuation and imbalance.

Sex hormones are not limited to estrogen and testosterone. There are three categories of hormones: 1) androgens that include testosterone and DHEA, 2) estrogens, and 3) progesterone. With so many players, a lot can happen. Beginning at puberty, roughly ages ten to 15, sex hormones become a game changer. In other words, they impact our daily lives. Sex hormones not only give us great pleasure but also bring forth headaches, both literally and figuratively. Keeping sex hormones "in line" before or during puberty often alleviates symptoms that can greatly impact lifestyle.

INDICATIONS OF POSSIBLE SEX HORMONE IMBALANCE

Chronic fatigue   Night sweats

Insomnia   Hot flashes

Weight gain   Restlessness

Moodiness/temper   Acne

Hair loss/gain   Bloating

Vaginal dryness/atrophy   Low libido

Period irregularity or stopping

ESTROGEN & PROGESTERONE

Many women (and some men with estrogen dominance) have a love-hate relationship with these hormones. Women want enough estrogen and progesterone to remain fertile, lustful, and youthful, but not so much as to become frenzied, angry, or incur an increased risk of cancer.

Estrogen is produced mostly in the ovaries, though it is also made in other places such as fat cells. This is worth repeating: estrogen is produced in fat cells. So, if you are experiencing estrogen dominance symptoms such as loss of sex drive, weight gain, headaches, fibroids, bloating, and are overweight, then it's advantageous to lose weight. Estrogen dominance often, though not always, goes hand in hand with a thyroid dysfunction, so it's important to distinguish between the two when you and your doctor work together to devise a wellness plan.

Estrogen receptors are in the skin, bone, breast tissue, uterine lining, and blood vessels. Receptors, like bouncers at a nightclub, "recognize" estrogen and allow it to enter into a cell where it manifests several functions. These include but are not limited to promoting skin thickness and elasticity for a more youthful look, relaxing blood vessels in the heart, enhancing bone strength, promoting healthier vaginal function, and providing a general sense of well-being.

When a woman's estrogen production wanes due to the natural process of aging, or due to a hysterectomy, she might experience sensations such as hot flashes, the inability to have a good night's sleep, night sweats, irregular periods, panic attacks, rapid aging, and/or mood swings. Though there is a common go-to list of perimenopausal and menopausal symptoms, these symptoms vary in frequency and intensity from woman to woman. At this time in life, it is wise to work with a doctor who sincerely sees *you* as an individual and not as just another menopausal woman. Technically, if there has been no menstrual cycle for twelve consecutive months, a woman has reached menopause, unless there is an underlying imbalance as to why her body is not menstruating. I have seen 20 and 30-something women go without cycles for 12 plus months due to extreme athletic training and/or disordered eating. If this is the case, you certainly want your doctor to address the reason for the imbalance and get the menstrual cycles flowing again. Lifestyle changes and healthy diets—particularly healthy fats, reviewing labs, and prescribing appropriate supplements or bioidentical hormones—can do this. If there has been a history of disordered eating, I request a therapist or psychologist be part of the wellness team.

Estrogen and progesterone are synergetic. Seldom should you address one and not the other. Progesterone is produced in the ovaries and integral in preparing the lining of the uterus for implantation of a fertilized egg and for maintenance of pregnancy. Sufficient progesterone is essential to becoming and remaining pregnant. If a woman experiences miscarriages, she will often be put on low-dose progesterone to increase the possibility of a full-term pregnancy.

When going through menopause, and at times perimenopause, many women seek hormonal supplementation to maintain a youthful, hormonal homeostasis. Very often at this time in life, the choice is made to start hormones (synthetic and/or bioidentical) for both physiological and mental improvements. This moves us into the subject of hormone replacement therapy (HRT).

HORMONE REPLACEMENT THERAPY: TO DO OR NOT TO DO?

With all the baby boomers becoming "aging boomers," HRT is discussed at dinner parties, on TV talk shows, and in sitcoms. HRT is the use of synthetic or natural hormones to make up for the lack of hormones the body no longer produces. It's not just women participating in this quest. Men, too, are interested in maintaining their youthfulness and cardiovascular and bone health. Lately, I have more men than women exploring the controversial HGH (human growth hormones) therapy which can cost thousands of dollars a month, in order to glean that mean and lean body.

Birth control pills are the most common form of HRT used by the medical establishment to address conditions such as acne, polycystic ovary syndrome (PCOS), premenstrual dysphoric disorder (PMDD), PMS, and menopausal symptoms. Hormone replacement therapy helps women and men with fertility, aging, and bone and cardiovascular health. A large scale, controlled 2002 trial from Denmark reported that healthy women taking combined HRT for ten years immediately after menopause had a reduced risk of heart disease and of dying from heart disease.[2]

Hormone replacement therapy can certainly be beneficial if given in the appropriate dosage and monitored annually by a physician with expertise in HRT. Women using HRT see improvement in mood, energy level, the ability to sleep, cardio-vascular health, vaginal health, and skin elasticity.

Integrative doctors tend to prescribe bioidentical HRT (compounds with the same chemical and molecular structure as hormones produced in the body) over synthetic

    2. Jennifer-Leigh Oprihory, "Danish Hormone Replacement Therapy Study Challenges HRT Risks," *Medill Reports Chicago*, October 10, 2012, accessed February 15, 2016, http://newsarchive.medill.northwestern.edu/chicago/news-208914.html.

versions, as do I. There appear to be fewer side effects with bioidentical formulas, potentially less residual harm, and patients like the idea of taking something that is more "natural." While there are arguments in favor of both forms of HRT, there is still plenty of research to be conducted on the pros and cons of all hormone replacement therapy. When deciding for yourself, choose to work with a compassionate healthcare professional knowledgeable about cutting-edge HRT, who also prescribes bioidentical hormones. Especially valuable is the choice of a doctor who will not shame you if *you choose* to use hormones. I stress *you choose*, because HRT is a significant lifestyle decision, and you should be the driver of this choice, not your physician, best friend, or significant other. It's a very personal decision that I honor, and I hope you do, too.

Once HRT becomes a part of your life, it is a good idea to have levels checked annually to make sure your dosage is correct and that your hormones are within normal ranges. I see too many female patients who remain on the same HRT dosage and/or blend for years without re-checking. You are not the same woman year-to-year, and your hormone levels are very likely to change just as you do.

TESTOSTERONE

Testosterone is the "male" hormone produced in the testes in men and the ovaries in women. It influences muscle and bone mass, red blood cell production, and sex drive. Levels naturally decrease with age, but other factors can cause testosterone production to drop, too, such as stress, chemo-therapy, radiation, hormonal disruption from chemicals in plastic containers, and in men, injury to the testicles and excessive bicycle riding. For males, lowered testosterone levels can cause increased moodiness, weight gain, loss of muscle mass, and diminished libido and sperm production.

I check the testosterone level in all my male patients with a blood draw or saliva test. If the test shows that levels are low, diet changes and supplementation can boost testosterone production and HRT is a possibility. If you begin taking testosterone, it's prudent to have your doctor monitor the level once within the first six months, and annually after that to make sure your body is processing the hormone and levels are not elevated. Excessive testosterone can accelerate aggression and risk-taking behavior.

In women, although circulating at much smaller levels, testosterone does contribute to healthy muscle and bone mass, a higher energy level, and overall wellness. I include testosterone testing when I check the sex hormones in my female patients, especially if they have low energy and low sex drive, an indication of low testosterone. Too high a level can explain issues such as increased anxiety, irritability, infertility, or polycystic ovarian syndrome (PCOS).

All too often, mainstream medicine ignores the testing of testosterone levels (especially in women) as if it has no role in our well-being. I beg to differ. It's well worth the time and financial investment to know what your testosterone levels are throughout different life phases. I recommend testing every year as a screening tool and as often as every six months if a patient is taking any kind of testosterone supplementation.

A key bit of information to remember is that testosterone is rarely the only issue in a hormone imbalance. It's well-advised to take a step back and look at other hormones, and indeed, the entire endocrine system, often zeroing in on the thyroid, adrenals, and glucose-insulin function.

DHEA

Dehydroepiandrosterone, or DHEA, is a hormone made from cholesterol and secreted by the adrenal glands in both men and women. It's a precursor to the sex hormones estrogen, progesterone, and testosterone. If DHEA is depleted, then very often the sex hormones are out of balance as well.

Extreme fatigue, decreased muscle mass and bone density, loss of libido, and sleep disturbance are some signs of low levels of DHEA (similar to adrenal fatigue). I rarely see high DHEA levels, but when I do, I request the patient cease all types of supplementation including DHEA, then re-test in two to three months. If the DHEA level remains high, then diagnostic imaging of the brain and/or adrenals is necessary to rule out tumor growth or abnormal swelling of the adrenals. If a tumor is found, it must be addressed by specialists such as an endocrinologist, oncologist, and surgeon to determine the best course of action.

Unlike testosterone and estrogen, DHEA is available over the counter, but I strongly advise patients not to attempt managing hormones on their own. Play it smart and work with an integrative doctor skilled in HRT to receive the optimum dosage for you. Have your DHEA level tested and then monitored one to two times a year to ensure that supplementation is still warranted.

MELATONIN

The word melatonin comes from the Greek root *melas,* meaning black or dark. Darkness stimulates the pineal gland to secrete the hormone melatonin, which can aid in better sleep. You can sometimes correct sleep problems by assisting the natural production of melatonin. To do this, make your bedroom as dark as possible. It's best to have no light visible, whether from nightlights, streetlights, the full moon, a TV screen, or the digital glow emanating from clocks, radios, security alarms, and phones. If darkness alone is an insufficient sleep aid, supplemental melatonin may help your body reach its natural rhythm.

Melatonin has a direct link to the "happy hormone," serotonin. Both affect not only sleep, but also mood, appetite, and a general sense of well-being. Melatonin is a powerful antioxidant, counteracting the damage of free radicals, and is often prescribed in higher doses (20 to 40 mg) to cancer patients. Though melatonin is a supplement available over the counter, work with an experienced healthcare professional to ensure the melatonin's quality and efficacy for your specific needs.

VITAMIN D

My patients are surprised when they learn that vitamin D is a hormone and not a vitamin. Vitamin D promotes bone formation and calcium absorption, and stimulates immune responses. It impacts thousands of genes throughout your body and may even inhibit cancer metastasis by reducing tumor secretion of enzymes that support growth. It's a complex hormone not to be overlooked!

We obtain inactive vitamin D from eating foods such as poultry, salmon, and eggs, and from UVB sunlight. The liver, kidneys, and skin then work in concert to make the inactive vitamin D active. This undertaking by the body is nothing short of miraculous, but it is often the case that not enough is produced to do an effective job. I find that over half of my patients need supplemental vitamin D during the fall and winter months when sunlight is at a minimum.

The question that is begging to be answered is why do so many of us have low amounts of vitamin D? Aging, lack of exposure to UVB sunlight, general inflammation, and gastrointestinal diseases like Celiac disease, gluten sensitivity, or poor digestion can all play a role in the deficiency. Some speculate that many of us are deficient because we shower with soap after being in the sun, washing the vitamin D from our skin. Perhaps it would pay to stay sweaty for a while and let all that good stuff soak in.

If lab results show that you do not have an optimum level of vitamin D, supplementation is advised. Choose the more natural and active vitamin D3 and not its synthetic counterpart, vitamin D2.

HCG

HCG (human chorionic gonadotropin) is the hormone responsible for the positive result in a pregnancy test. I mention it not because it's integral to balancing hormones, but because it is used in a popular hormone weight loss diet for both women and men—the HCG diet. The theory behind this diet is that HCG allows the body to shed fat, not muscle tissue, during the diet. Most patients lose between a half a pound and a pound per day by injecting or ingesting HCG and eating the prescribed foods. The real work, and real benefit, comes from integrating the healthful diet into your lifestyle once you stop taking the hormone. What seems so successful for patients who have used the HCG diet is the very noticeable ten to thirty pounds lost in an acceptable and rewarding timespan. This progress provides the hope and motivation needed to continue the new eating habits. And that's the trick—the diet becomes not a one-time venture, but a new way of living.

If you are interested in pursuing the HCG diet, it is not available over the counter. A prescription is needed.

HELP YOUR HORMONES AND THEY WILL HELP YOU

Hormones are messengers delivering essential life-giving information to individual cells and to systems of the body. We need to hone our listening skills and pay close attention when they call out to us.

WHEN HORMONES ARE IN BALANCE—TUNED UP—LIFE IS MORE IN HARMONY.

The endocrine system is like an orchestra, and you (with the guidance of your licensed health-care professional) need to be able to hear the music and then distinguish the drumbeat from the violins and the oboes. Each hormone has a distinctive part to play and yet works in unison with the others. When hormones are in balance—tuned up—life is more in harmony.

CHAPTER 8 HEALTH RESOLUTIONS

Have you had your hormone levels checked recently? Ever? If not, whether you are male or female, please check off the following:

1. I, ——————————————————————,
    will make an appointment with my doctor and ask her to run the following labs: vitamin D, DHEA, estrogen (estradiol), progesterone, free and total testosterone, and cortisol levels via saliva samples gathered throughout the day.

2. I will review the results in detail with my doctor.

3. If HRT is warranted, I will collaborate with my doctor to find the right product and dosage for me.

Upon fulfilling this chapter's Health Resolutions, if your lab results are all within the normal range, be thankful. It is also great to know your personal "normal," so you have a baseline for future diagnoses.

CHAPTER 9

Labs: The Inside Scoop

Laboratory tests (labs) are often the exact tool needed to eliminate the guesswork when diagnosing a condition. Labs reveal the tip of the iceberg, the first bit of information needed, to embark on a more direct path toward health. With enlightening data provided by lab work, you and your licensed healthcare professional can dig deeper and discover the underlying cause of your less-than-optimum state of health.

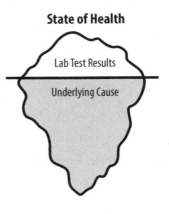

The information provided in this chapter is a lab test primer. The intent is to provide rudimentary knowledge that should enable you to become more in charge of your own well-being.

When you have your blood drawn, pee in a cup, poop into a plastic container, spit into a vial, or any other lovely variation of collecting bodily specimens, test results provide valuable clues as to what's going on in your body. Labs provide:

- a baseline of what your body's chemistry is like when it is working well,

- a way to detect trends unique to your body and/or time in life,

- a clue to discovering the root cause of what is bothering you, and

- a means to monitoring progress and wellness plan effectiveness.

Though lab tests can often cost hundreds of dollars out of network, they most often pay for themselves. For example, let's say you have been treated repeatedly for chronic sinus infections over the past two years. You've paid for numerous rounds of antibiotics and over-the-counter supplements and still missed several days of work because you felt horrible. Frustrated, you try a new integrated physician who runs a few specifically targeted labs, and immediately it's discovered your sinus infection is fungal, not bacterial. This explains why the antibiotics never worked and suggests another form of treatment is needed. All that money spent prior to the alternative doctor's lab tests was a waste.

The Health Revolution is about you being empowered so you can take more initiative regarding your health. Labs very often provide the info needed to do just that. The tricky part is making sure your doctor dedicates sufficient time to thoroughly discuss your test results so that you understand what's happening "below the surface." *Always* request copies of your labs—every time—and create your own lab test folder at home, digital or hardcopy. That way you are in control and not at the mercy of some medical records person in a cubicle somewhere. Having current lab test results at your fingertips proves useful for additional medical consultations or in the case of a medical emergency.

ALWAYS REQUEST COPIES OF YOUR LABS.

There are hundreds of possible lab tests to run. I have codified the labs I order repeatedly into six categories:

1. Baseline

2. Second Tier Baseline

3. Sex Hormone

4. Inflammation Markers

5. Viral and Fungal

6. Gut Health

The category (ies) I recommend to a patient depends upon the individual's health concerns and history. All these tests provide the patient, and me, with solid information from which we can create a wellness plan, monitor progress, and determine if a referral to a specialized healthcare professional is required.

#1. BASELINE LABS

No matter your age, gender, or in most cases the state of your health, there are labs I order every year or at the most every two years for my patients. These baseline labs provide a rudimentary look at the status of your body's well-being. Here are the labs I consider baseline.

Complete Blood Count (CBC) provides a count of the red and white blood cells in a sample of your blood. A CBC can indicate whether or not your body is fighting infection or is anemic. If anemia is discovered, this test will further delineate if it is due to an iron deficiency or a B12 deficiency.

Comprehensive Metabolic Panel (CMP) provides information on liver and kidney functions such as filtration rate and inflammatory responses, as well as the levels of common electrolytes like calcium, potassium, sodium, and chloride.

Vitamin D lab work provides us with the level of vitamin D in the blood. This hormone augments bone production and also plays a crucial role in the immune system. Many of us are deficient in vitamin D and a blood test can indicate if supplementation is needed.

A1C test results reflect an average blood sugar level for the past ninety days, not just the day of your blood draw as a glucose test would. This test is used to diagnose diabetes and monitor treatment success, as well as to track how a person is doing with dietary goals. If the A1C level begins to creep upward, and it is addressed, there's a great chance of preventing diabetes through diet, health education, and supplementation. If I can prevent even one person from going down the diabetes road, then I am one happy doctor.

Insulin labs disclose the amount of insulin produced by specialized beta cells in the pancreas. This blood test is often ordered with A1C to determine if a person is insulin resistant, pre-diabetic, or diabetic. It can also rule out suspected pancreatic tumors. Insulin tests can determine how much insulin in the blood the body produces and how much is made by medication.

A **Lipid Panel** indicates cholesterol and triglyceride levels. Triglycerides are basically stored fats. Cholesterol is a fatty substance found on every cell on your body, and your body needs just enough of it to function properly. In order to obtain an accurate test result, you must fast for at least twelve hours before the blood test. Elevated results suggest diet and lifestyle changes are necessary.

Too many people are put on cholesterol lowering medications without being educated on how to lower levels more naturally.

Thyroid Stimulating Hormone (TSH) labs depict how well the pituitary gland is communicating with the thyroid. This test can help detect if a patient is dealing with hypothyroidism, hyperthyroidism, Hashimoto's disease, or thyroid cancer.

Free T3 and Free T4 measures the thyroid hormones that are available (free to use) for metabolism. In a nutshell, T4 is converted to T3 and some of the cofactors used in this conversion are: selenium, iodine, B6, magnesium, and glutathione. Your body needs these hormones to regulate temperature, weight, and metabolism.

A PAP (Papanicolaou) Test and Vaginal Swab should be conducted every one or two years depending on a woman's age, health risk, and sexual activity. A vaginal swab is different than a PAP test. A PAP examines the cervical cells looking for Human Papillomavirus (HPV), precancerous cells, or cancer, while a vaginal swab determines bacterial infections, yeast overgrowth, or STDs (sexual transmitted diseases). Vaginal infections or overgrowths can be asymptomatic, so it's advisable to be tested if you are sexually active and/or experiencing any abnormal discharge, itching, or discomfort. Infections love dark warm places and the vaginal cavity is a place for them to flourish.

A **mammogram** is an X-ray of the breasts most often used to detect cancer in women. Men, too, can develop breast cancer and should seek a doctor's consultation upon noticing pain, a lump, or swelling in the breast or discharge from the nipple. I recommend mammograms for women starting at the age of 50 and then having one every two years, unless there is a specific reason to screen more frequently such as a personal or familial history of breast cancer. A manual breast exam should be conducted yearly at the time of a physical, and monthly at home. Some women choose thermography (measurement of temperature or infrared radiation) over mammography, but this screening tool is not currently accepted by mainstream medicine and is often not reimbursed by insurance companies. I have little experience with thermography, and for that reason, refer patients interested in this choice to a specialist. As for tissue biopsies, I suggest seeking a second opinion before agreeing to this invasive procedure. Radiologists quickly recommend this procedure when there are at times appropriate alternatives, such as "vigilantly watch and wait," altering the diet, checking hormone levels, and running more labs. No patient or healthcare professional wants to miss a tumor, but all too often doctors act aggressively, stressing the immediate need for a biopsy with every abnormal finding.

Prostate-Specific Antigen (PSA) measures the amount of PSA in the blood of males. An antigen, in simple words, is any substance that causes the immune system to produce antibodies. This lab should be conducted every one or two years depending on a man's age, health risk, and sexual activity. Common symptoms that may warrant a PSA lab test are difficulty urinating, a full sensation in the rectum, and pain or discomfort with orgasm.

There is a fair amount of controversy regarding whether or not a PSA lab result is an accurate screening tool for prostate health, BPH (benign prostate hyperplasia), infection, or cancer. Even so, it is known that the higher the PSA value, the higher the probability these negative conditions exist. I recommend obtaining a baseline PSA value beginning at the age of 45 and watching for trends yearly. Results over 3.50 ng/ml, even without symptoms, warrant a re-check every twelve months, and I refer such patients with symptoms to an integrative urologist. Prostate cancer, of course, should be the first condition to consider if the test reveals abnormal values. If prostate cancer is diagnosed, I recommend two to three opinions before any surgery, chemotherapy, and radiation, and when merited, to "watch and wait." If one is interested in reading more on the topic, the book *Thrive Don't Only Survive! Dr. Geo's Guide to Living Your Best Life Before and After Prostate Cancer* by Dr. Geo Espinosa with Mathew Solan offers invaluable lifestyle information for not only prostate patients, but also their partners. A reputable online resource is the website Harvardprostateknowledge.org.

#2. SECOND TIER BASELINE LABS

After baseline labs are completed, if further investigation is warranted in order to create a wellness plan, there are additional labs I may suggest. Note that I do not order all these labs indiscriminately. Labs are ordered contingent upon each individual's health status.

> **Thyroid antibodies (Anti-TPO & TGAb)** blood tests can provide an accurate diagnosis for Hashimoto's disease, an autoimmune condition that affects the thyroid. The first antibody, anti-TPO, initiates inflammation on the thyroid follicles. The second antibody, TGAb, attacks the key protein in the thyroid gland, thyroglobulin. I test for antibodies when the baseline thyroid labs are abnormal or the patient continues to report symptoms of a thyroid disorder even if prior labs are in or near normal ranges. It's crucial to know whether or not a patient is producing thyroid antibodies so a wellness plan can be put into place that will help prevent further damage to the thyroid. If left unchecked, these antibodies often lead to thyroid removal or ablation, which puts a patient on thyroid medication for life.
>
> **Thyroid Stimulating Immunoglobulin (TSI)** is ordered as an additional test to rule out Graves' disease, an autoimmune condition related to hyperthyroidism.

Vitamin B12 and Folic Acid levels are checked if the CBC blood test is abnormal and/or if the patient is experiencing miscarriages, low energy, headaches, nerve pain, poor memory, or other neurological symptoms.

Methylmalonic Acid (MMA) is a compound that reacts with vitamin B12 to create energy. It's a more sensitive test than a B12 test alone. I tend to order it when I see B12 at a low level or as a way to monitor the effectiveness of a wellness plan.

Ferritin is tested if the CBC result is abnormal and indicates further investigation of iron storage. Ferritin levels reflect how well the body is storing iron. Too little ferritin can indicate iron deficient anemia, a small internal bleed, or inflammatory conditions causing malabsorption of nutrients. High levels can lead to joint pain, liver disease, or organ failure, and may indicate hereditary hemochromatosis. Hemochromatosis is a condition in which the body absorbs too much iron from food and stores it in organs. This can lead to life-threatening conditions such as diabetes, liver disease, and heart problems.

C-Peptide lab tests reflect the amount of insulin produced by the pancreas only and do not take into account levels produced by medication. This lab allows us to determine how well the pancreas is or is not producing insulin and can direct the creation of appropriate wellness plans with pre-diabetic and diabetic patients.

#3. SEX HORMONE LABS

All sex hormones can be tested via blood or saliva. I recommend having these tests run every two to three years, or every six to 12 months if the patient is on hormone replacement therapy of any kind. If a woman is still menstruating, saliva samples should be collected every three to five days throughout the month. Most patients don't find it convenient to spit into vials over an entire month, so a one-time blood test is often the more desirable choice. A post-menopausal woman may provide just one saliva sample since there isn't much hormonal fluctuation occurring. Unfortunately, many of the sex hormone lab tests, especially saliva, typically are not covered by insurance. (Time to change the system.)

> **Estrogen** saliva tests can be used to measure all three estrogens: E1 (Estrone), E2 (Estradiol), and E3 (Estriol), which provides detailed information for prescribing hormone replacement therapy. A blood test most often determines the level of E2 (Estradiol) only, E2 being the most active estrogen produced by the ovaries and commonly used in estrogen replacement therapy along with E3 (Estriol).

> **Progesterone** levels are equally important to evaluate as this hormone works synergistically with estrogen. Progesterone can be tested via saliva or a blood draw as well. Often a woman might start hormone therapy with only a progesterone cream or pill to help alleviate

what is known as "estrogen dominance." Estrogen dominance can present symptoms such as anxiety, loss of sex drive, headaches, fatigue, hypoglycemia, painful intercourse, bloating, acne, and menstrual cycles lasting longer than the normal 5-8 days or with excessive bleeding, which may cause anemia.

Testosterone is present in both men and women. It plays a role in building muscle mass, reducing fat, improving mood, and increasing energy, sex drive, concentration, and a sense of well-being. Levels vary depending on gender and age and may be tested via saliva or a blood draw. It's best to order both free and total testosterone to get a more complete picture of testosterone and how it is working with you or against you.

Cortisol levels are best determined from saliva or urine samples taken throughout the day. When samples are taken morning, noon, early evening, and after midnight, a pattern can be detected and compared to what a normal rise and fall would be. Desired results will show cortisol levels that are high in the morning (energetic) and decreasing gradually throughout the day (tired in the evening). This lab information helps determine which lifestyle changes, supplements, and herbs to implement.

DHEA is produced in the adrenal glands and is interactive with the other sex hormones. Low levels of DHEA may cause such symptoms as low energy, sleep loss, and

loss of libido. Many patients come to me having chosen to take over-the-counter DHEA with or without
the guidance of a licensed healthcare professional. This
is hormone replacement therapy, and annual testing
should be emphasized to determine if supplementation
is indeed necessary and to provide a marker with which
to determine future treatment. If DHEA is depleted,
then very often the sex hormones are out of balance.

AN HRT SUCCESS STORY

One of my patients recently decided to try hormone replacement therapy after two years of menopausal symptoms. She
seldom had a day without feeling frustrated because of low
energy, non-existent libido, forgetfulness, and endless hot
flashes. We tested her hormones and discovered she was
low in estrogen, progesterone, and DHEA. Her liver and
thyroid functions were normal as was her cholesterol level.
With this data in hand, I recommended a compounding
pharmacy that blended a hormone cream specifically for
her. The cream contained bioidentical estrogens, progesterone, and DHEA. Within weeks of applying this cream, she
was energetic and felt "more like herself." After six months,
we rechecked her levels to ensure her body was utilizing
the hormones correctly. High hormone levels can lead to a
return of the original symptoms or menstrual cycles, aches,
sore joints, liver inflammation, bloating, mood swings, and
potentially cancer. Her follow-up labs indicated normal,

healthy levels. This, accompanied by improved libido and sleep, the rare hot flash, and the fact that she looked great, was sufficient evidence for her to continue HRT.

#4. INFLAMMATORY MARKERS

"Inflammation, inflammation, inflammation" tout the medical journals and diet books of late. Along with genetics, inflammation is the hot medical topic of the 21st century, largely due to the fact that we still do not completely understand it. Signs and symptoms include, but are by no means limited to, swollen tissues, joint pain, chronic pain, fatigue, headaches, depression, poor eyesight, bloating, and weight gain or loss.

Inflammation occurs when the body attempts to protect itself from harmful agents. It's the body's first endeavor to heal after assault from an undesirable intruder such as an infection. Chronic inflammation occurs when the body is unable to overcome the effects of the injuring agent. It can burn out of control and be the precursor to diseases such as heart disease and cancer.[1] If you're experiencing chronic aches and pains, digestive issues, diabetes, heart disease, or cancer, it's beneficial to have inflammatory marker testing done to determine your baseline and monitor and treat accordingly. Love yourself by changing your diet, moving your body, and supplementing properly with guidance

1. Gary Stix, "A Malignant Flame," *Scientific American*, July 2007, accessed August 21, 2016, http://www.scientificamerican.com/article/a-malignant-flame/.

from a licensed healthcare professional. Three to 12 months later, retest and see if the inflammation has decreased. Also pay close attention to how you feel, because as inflammation is addressed, symptoms melt away one by one and you may suddenly realize that you're feeling significantly better. There are six labs that provide inflammation data that can be used to craft treatment goals and monitor progress along with reported symptoms:

Insulin-like Growth Factor 1 (IGF-1) is necessary for proper growth in children, but studies of men and women over 40 raise the possibility that IGF-1 contributes to the growth of tumors (cancer) especially in the colon, prostate, and breasts.[2] Prominent universities such as Harvard and Boston University are conducting studies with IGF-1 and its role in regard to chronic inflammation and cancer.

Lactate Dehydrogenase or Lactic Acid Dehydrogenase (LDH or LD) is an enzyme found in almost all of the body's cells. It's released from distressed cells into the blood plasma and can be a general indicator of tissue and cellular damage. Extreme athletes and folks dealing with inflammatory conditions in the body often have higher levels of LDH.

2. William J. Cromie, "Growth Factor Raises Cancer Risk," *The Harvard University Gazette*, April 22, 1999, accessed February 15, 2016, http://news.harvard.edu/gazette/1999/04.22/igf1.story.html.

C-reactive protein (CRP) is used to detect inflammation when tissue injury or infection is suspected. This test can also help evaluate the risk of developing coronary heart disease.

Sed Rate (ESR) is a blood test that often confirms inflammation is present. It's a general test, and not diagnostic to a specific disease. ESR rate measures the distance red blood cells fall into a test tube in an hour. Less than 15 mm per hour is ideal. Because ESR is not specific, it is essential to look at all the inflammatory markers to hone in on a diagnosis. Sed Rate helps you and your integrative doctor monitor the progress of your wellness plan.

Homocysteine is an amino acid and by-product of protein metabolism. When present in high concentrations as determined by a blood test, it has been linked to an increased risk of heart attack and stroke. A few contributors to an increase in homocysteine levels are lack of B vitamins in the diet, inflammation, stress, and genetic mutations. The ideal range is 4-10 umol/L, but I often see patients with chronic inflammation levels at 20-80 umol/L.

TGF Beta-1 (Transforming Growth Factor Beta-1) is a protein found throughout the body that helps control the growth, division, and proliferation of cells. Neurological and autoimmune issues, as well as numbness and tingling of toes and fingers, go hand-in-hand with high TGF Beta-1 results. High value test results also warrant further testing for exposure to mold.

#5. VIRAL AND FUNGAL LABS

Viruses can be covert disruptors to health. You would be surprised how many of my patients have had underlying viral infections and were unaware of them. Over time, untamed viral and fungal infections can lead to chronic fatigue and a long list of debilitating symptoms, such as unexplained numbness and tingling of extremities, chronic headaches and/or colds, muscle aches, and low stamina. Viral and fungal IgG blood tests determine the levels and presence of IgG antibodies, which indicate whether or not a patient has been exposed to a virus or fungus. Elevated IgG values demand a rigorous wellness plan. When on such a recovery plan, retesting after six months or a year is needed to ensure IgG antibody values are decreasing.

Herpes Simplex (HSV-1, HSV-2) IgG blood tests search for antibodies that indicate exposure to the specific herpes viruses HSV-1 and HSV-2. Most people know about these two herpes viruses: HSV-1, appearing as the common cold sore on facial lips, and HSV-2, which appears on the genitals, but there are numerous herpes viruses that can have a detrimental impact on health. IgG blood tests need to be run for each specific herpes virus. Patients with chronic fatigue and pain, paralysis, random numbness, tingling of the fingers and toes, or a history of oral herpes, genital herpes, or shingles outbreaks should consider testing.

EBV (Epstein-Barr Virus, HSV 4) IgG blood tests search for antibodies that indicate exposure to the Epstein-Barr virus. EBV is what causes the "kissing disease"—mononucleosis—and it, too, is in the herpes family. EBV is also linked to numerous cancers and autoimmune conditions.

CMV (Cytomegalovirus, HSV 5) IgG blood tests search for antibodies that indicate exposure to the Cytomegalovirus. CMV is linked to some pneumonias and salivary gland conditions, as well as mononucleosis, but is not directly responsible for it like EBV. If blood tests for either Herpes Simplex, EBV, or CMV reveal high levels, the wellness plan can weigh heavily on antiviral herbs and supplements, such as lemon balm, licorice, ginger, garlic, osha root, and olive leaf, as well as basic immune support provided by medical mushrooms, hydrotherapy, diet, and proper rest.

Candida IgG blood tests search for antibodies that indicate exposure to candida (a fungus). Often, chronic sinus, ear, vaginal, and oral infections are fungal and not viral or bacterial. If you have taken numerous rounds of antibiotics for an infection without treatment success, then it's time to rule out a fungal infection with both a culture and this blood test.

#6. GUT HEALTH LABS

Doctor's Data Comprehensive Stool Analysis measures the unique ribosomal protein fingerprints of microorganisms from three different bowel movements. It is able to identify over 1,200 species of bacteria and yeast, and the Cleveland Clinic ranked it in the *Top 10 Medical Innovations* list. Not only does this test reveal what normal and abnormal bacteria and yeast are present, it also shows common inflammatory markers, stool pH and secretory IgA (SIgA), which is a marker of gut mucosal barrier integrity and immunity. It's a comprehensive test not to be ignored with any type of gut imbalance.

Genova's Comprehensive Organic Acids Profile looks for certain organic acids that are by-products of bacterial and fungal metabolism. These can indicate bacterial or fungal overgrowth in the GI tract. In addition to gut health, these organic acids are also by-products of cellular metabolism and provide insight on how well metabolic cycles of the body are working. For each of these metabolic cycles, specific enzymes are needed. In turn, the enzymes require particular nutrients to function properly. If the body is deficient in the required nutrient, the metabolic cycle will not complete, resulting in a buildup of the organic acid spilling into the urine sample. Once you know what the nutritional deficiency is, you can work on providing the body with the needed nutrients. This urine test offers information on detoxification pathways, general metabolism, neurotransmitter breakdown, cellular energy production, and fatty acid and carbohydrate metabolism. For example, a common organic acid marker is methylmalonic acid (MMA), which indicates a vitamin B12 deficiency more accurately than only measuring B12 levels in the blood. A vitamin B12 deficiency can be corrected by taking B12 orally or by receiving intramuscular injections of B12 for three to six months, and then reassessing how the body is both using and storing B12. Got Vitamin B12 clinics (Gotvitaminb12.com) in California and Colorado are a great resource for easy and affordable B12 injections.

Genova's SIBO Breath Test is prudent to run if small intestinal bacterial overgrowth (SIBO) is suspected. There is potential for both false positives and false negatives, so do not rely on SIBO breath test results alone. When this test is combined with Genova's Comprehensive Organic Acids Profile and Doctor's Data Comprehensive Stool Analysis, a wealth of data is provided for better assessing the status of one's gut health.

LABS AT-A-GLANCE

Baseline			
Lab Test	*Frequency*	*Type*	*Optimal Ranges*
CBC	Annually	Blood	Optimal RBC count is 4.25-5.25, WBC 5.5-8.5, hematocrit 85+/- 3 with no indication of infection
CMP	Annually	Blood	Each individual test within a normal range
Vitamin D	Annually	Blood	50-75 ng/ml
A1C	1-4 times/ year	Blood	< 5.25 %
Insulin	1-4 times/ year	Blood	AM fasting <5 No fasting <9-12
Lipid Panel	Annually	Blood	Cholesterol <220, triglycerides half of cholesterol, triglycerides equal to HDL, HDL > 65, LDL < 95

Lab Test	Frequency	Type	Optimal Ranges
TSH	Annually	Blood	0.75-2.25 mIU/L
Free T3 & Free T4	Annually with TSH	Blood	High end of the normal range
PAP/Vaginal Swab	1 year or every other year contingent on age and history	Exam & Swab	Normal cervical cells/ no abnormal bacteria or Candida, vaginal pH 3.5-4.5
Mammogram	Every 2 years after the age of 50, unless otherwise indicated	X-ray	Normal tissue
PSA	Annually after the age of 45	Blood	< 3.50 ng/ml
Second Tier Baseline			
Anti-TPO & TGAb	As needed	Blood	< 1:100 IU/ml
TSI	As needed	Blood	< 1.3 TSI index
B12	If anemia is suspected	Blood	> 600 pg/ml

Lab Test	Frequency	Type	Optimal Ranges
Folic acid	If anemia is suspected	Blood	14-18 ng/ml
MMA	If B12 deficient and/or anemia is suspected	Blood	At or lower than the normal range, as specified by each individual laboratory
Ferritin	If anemia is suspected	Blood	Women > 50 and < 150 Men > 50 and < 225
C-peptide	If type 2 diabetic	Blood	Yearly to monitor pancreatic function and need for insulin
Sex Hormones			
Estrogen	1 year	Blood or Saliva	Varies per individual, type of test, and timing
Progesterone	1 year	Blood or Saliva	Varies per individual, type of test, and timing
Free and Total Testosterone	1 year	Blood or Saliva	Varies per individual, type of test, and timing

Lab Test	Frequency	Type	Optimal Ranges
Cortisol	1-4 years	Saliva	Elevated in the morning and lower in the evening
DHEA	1-4 years	Blood or Saliva	At the high end of the normal range
Inflammatory Markers			
IGF-1	Varies with diagnosis	Blood	<100 mg/L
LDH/LD	Varies with diagnosis	Blood	<150 u/L
CRP	Varies with diagnosis	Blood	<1.0 mg/L
Sed Rate (ESR)	Varies with diagnosis	Blood	<15 mm/hr
Homocysteine	Varies with diagnosis	Blood	4-10 umol/L
TGF Beta-1	Varies with diagnosis	Blood	Normal range < 2380 pg/ml
Viral and Fungal			
HSV-1 IgG & HSV-2 IgG	Once, then monitor as needed	Blood	Negative range

Lab Test	Frequency	Type	Optimal Ranges
EBV (HSV-4) IgG	Once, then monitor as needed	Blood	Negative range
CMV (HSV-5) IgG	Once, then monitor as needed	Blood	Negative range
Candida IgG	Once, then monitor as needed	Blood	Negative range
Gut Health Labs			
Doctor's Data Comprehensive Stool Analysis	As needed with unresolved digestive conditions	Stool	Normal ranges with all results
Genova's Comprehensive Organic Acids Profile	As needed with unresolved chronic medical conditions	Urine	Normal ranges with all results
Genova's SIBO Breath Test	As needed to rule out SIBO and to monitor wellness plan effectiveness	Breath	Negative range

LAB TEST SUMMARY

Laboratory tests are just one of the eight guidelines that will keep you on a trajectory toward health and away from disease. Too often patients fear labs and avoid them. If this describes you, reframe the reason you are obtaining labs, as the purpose should be to understand more precisely what is happening inside your body. Labs render insight into your unique biochemical makeup. I invite you to step up to the plate, know your biochemistry, and from that point, develop a wellness plan with your doctor that will deliver health.

CHAPTER 9 HEALTH RESOLUTION

Have you been dealing with a persistent health issue? Have you avoided getting a physical exam for at least two years? If you answered "yes" to either or both of these questions, please make an appointment with an integrative doctor you trust, who will work with you as a partner in designing your wellness plan. Request recommended labs (you can use my baseline list to start), and then thoroughly discuss the results with your doctor. Learn how you can improve your lab results and overall health in the next three, six, and

LET THE INFORMATION GLEANED FROM LAB TESTS EMPOWER YOU, NOT SCARE YOU.

twelve months. What assistance can your doctor provide, other than medication, to fulfill your health goals?

I will go to my doctor and have lab work done by _____. If my doctor seems less than interested, I will find another doctor. This is a promise I am making to myself and keeping!

Let the information gleaned from lab tests empower you, not scare you.

CHAPTER 10

The Lost Art of Relaxing

What do you do in your daily life to chill out, slow down, breathe, or relax? The sad truth is that most Americans have a never-ending to-do list, and it seldom, if ever, includes time for relaxation. This constant going and doing is a substantial contributor to our individual and collective ill health. All too often, I hear patients, friends, and family say, "I'm exhausted and I don't know how to slow down." It's helpful to be aware that it's not so much the amount or type of stress we have, but *how we react to it* that determines our state of health and emotional well-being. After a particularly stressful day, do you meditate, take a walk, have a drink(s), or stare at the TV?

Stress can come from a traumatic experience or a long-standing, less-than-desirable situation. Death of a loved one, injury, trouble at work, loss of a job, divorce, disease, and teenagers—can all cause stress. Generalized fears, too, have a direct impact on the body and mind. Patients very often share with me the fear of not having enough money, despite the amount they have. Wealthy patients talk about this concern as well as those who don't know how next month's rent is going to be paid. Fears such as running out of money can create hours of mind chatter. If we can quiet the chatter, we will be more in the moment, calmer, and more content with our lives.

I often discuss with patients the give-and-take relationship between time, money, and health. Which one of the three would you take more of if you could choose only one?

> BUSY IS GOOD.
> BUSY IS GOD.
> BUSY STOPS US
> FROM...THINKING
> AND FEELING.

The majority choose time—more time to relax, to enjoy friends and family, and less time worrying. I like to call this time "getting para," referring to the parasympathetic nervous system, which is the state our body enters when we "rest and digest." It is the opposite of the survival-based sympathetic nervous system that runs the show when we're constantly stressed or "running from the tiger": our boss, a rough relationship, or our endless things-to-do list.

Somewhere in our modern day evolution, we have begun to equate busy with value. Busy is good. Busy is God. Busy stops us from...thinking and feeling. And that is almost exactly my point. We can't raise a revolution without thinking and feeling passionate about the cause, can we?

Prominent universities such as UC-San Francisco, Stanford, and Harvard pour millions of dollars into parasympathetic research and its importance in medicine and healing.[1] Integrative physicians understand existing in the parasympathetic nervous system is a vital part in the healing process and not just a New Age hypothesis. Everyone can benefit from getting para from time to time. Normalizing blood pressure and lowering cortisol levels is possible with a daily meditation practice. The power of prayer has its place in reducing stress, as does the clinical application of herbs and supplements (passionflower, chamomile, valerian, kava-kava, and magnesium, to name a few) that promote a more parasympathetic state. If you were given a choice between taking a medication with a long list of side effects to lower your blood pressure or leaning on the art of meditation for 15 minutes a day, which would you prefer?

Stress can be the precursor to hair loss, weight gain, lack of libido, insomnia, colitis, and cancer. Cortisol, released by the adrenal glands, plays a leading role in regard to stress. Elevated cortisol, influenced by our over-active, sympathetic lifestyles, disrupts digestion by impeding

1. "Mindfulness Meditation Could Lower Levels of Cortisol, The Stress Hormone," *The Huffington Post*, Huffpost Healthy Living, 3/31/2013, accessed 2/8/2016, http://www.huffingtonpost.com/2013/03/31/mindfulness-meditation-cortisol-stress-levels_n_2965197.html.

Brigid Schulte, "Harvard neuroscientist: Meditation not only reduces stress, here's how it changes your brain," *The Washington Post*, 5/26/2015, accessed February 9, 2016, https://www.washingtonpost.com/news/inspired-life/wp/2015/05/26/harvard-neuroscientist-meditation-not-only-reduces-stress-it-literally-changes-your-brain/.

absorption of digestive enzymes and nutrients. It also pre-
vents a good night's sleep and wreaks havoc on the glucose-
insulin relationship, creating mood swings and cravings
for carbohydrates. Excessive cortisol also suppresses the
immune system, and as a result, impairs the body's ability
to fight seasonal allergies, colds, or infections.

When you are under stress, a variety of things can go
wrong. Does your back go out? Do you have migraine
headaches, acid reflux, break out with acne, or do you reach
for the cookie jar? In my case, my allergies kick in with
swollen eyes and sneezing, often accompanied by a bloated
belly. We can counteract many of these unpleasant conditions if we learn to slow down and relax.

Entering into a para state by curling up with a good
book or sharing a leisurely meal with friends allows the
mind, body, and soul time to rejuvenate, which in turn
helps us live in our hectic, techno, tail-chasing world.
Taking a time-out is not only for two-year-olds. Keeping
calm is the new cool these days. I invite you to create more
para in your life to rejuvenate and connect with self, others,
and your surroundings.

HOW TO GET MORE PARA

Drugs and alcohol are often used as de-stressors. Eventually,
this can lead to a shaky lifestyle, often rendering an individual unable to cope during life's difficult times. To find
a substitute for a few martinis or beers after work, think

about what relaxes your shoulders and connects you with the world in a positive way, without any negative effects on the body, mind, or spirit. For each of us there exists unique, satisfying, and healthful ways to move from the sympathetic state to one that is more parasympathetic. Here are some pleasurable and restorative activities (in no particular order) to consider:

WAYS TO "GET PARA"

Meditation/prayer

Breathwork

12-48 hour break from technology (phone, computer, TV)

Massage

Chiropractic adjustments

Sipping tea

Rest—sleeping, napping, and lounging

Reading a book

Playing an instrument/singing

Journaling

Crossword puzzles, jigsaw puzzles, card and board games

Walking in nature, walking a labyrinth, or with a dog

Gardening

Bird watching

Cooking, baking, canning

Watching the sunset/sunrise or moon rise or fall

Soaking in hot springs

Orgasm (snuck that one in)

Vacationing/abandoning the daily routine

Hobbies: knitting, scrapbooking, stamp collecting

Dining leisurely with others

Movement/yoga/martial arts

Exercise that is fun and inspiring

Let's look at a few options that can be especially helpful in relieving stress, but are too readily dismissed or frequently not even considered.

MEDITATION

As mentioned earlier, science is backing up the benefits of the ancient practice of meditation. Researchers at Johns Hopkins University in Baltimore, Maryland, have collated 47 well-designed scientific studies strongly suggesting that mindfulness meditation can help ease psychological stresses such as anxiety, depression, and pain.[2] It's not just for monks, yogis, and sages anymore. In fact, some public school systems are now integrating meditation into their

IF YOU DON'T THINK MEDITATION IS FOR YOU, OR THAT YOU CAN'T SIT STILL... MEDITATION IS PROBABLY FOR YOU!

---

2. Madhav Goyal, MD, MPH; Sonal Singh, MD, MPH; Erica M. S. Sibinga, MD, MHS; Neda F. Gould, PhD; Anastasia Rowland-Seymour, MD; Ritu Sharma, BSc; Zackary Berger, MD, PhD; Dana Sleicher, MS, MPH; David D. Maron, MHS; Hasan M. Shihab, MBChB, MPH; Padmini D. Ranasinghe, MD, MPH; Shauna Linn, BA; Shonali Saha, MD; Eric B. Bass, MD, MPH; Jennifer A. Haythornthwaite, PhD, "Meditation Programs for Psychological Stress and Well-Being: A Systematic Review and Meta-analysis," *JAMA Intern Med.* 2014;174(3):357-368, accessed June 8, 2016, http://archinte.jamanetwork.com/article.aspx?articleid=1809754.

daily curriculum to help students deal with "violence and the trauma and the stress of everyday life."[3]

Many Americans believe meditation is attached to a certain religion or belief system, but it can be a non-denominational practice from which any person can benefit. Meditation can take on many forms, and it is associated with relaxation, serenity, stilling the mind, developing compassion and forgiveness, and simply "being." It can be done while sitting still or while moving, as in walking a labyrinth. Quietly watching the birds splashing in the birdbath can be considered a form of meditation. My dad, for example, watches and feeds his chipmunks every morning. If feeding chipmunks is not for you, then look for meditation classes. They are offered across the country, so ask around, or search on the Internet. You can find many books, guided audio meditations, and YouTube videos on how to begin. Oprah Winfrey and Deepak Chopra have created excellent 21-day meditation challenges that can connect you to thousands of people around the world (Chopracentermeditation.com). It's a powerful para moment when you realize so many human beings are purposefully connecting to love at the same time. If you don't think meditation is for you, or that you can't sit still...meditation is probably for you!

3. San Francisco Schools Transformed by the Power of Meditation, *NBC Nightly News*, Jan 1, 2015, accessed February 9, 2016, http://www.nbcnews.com/nightly-news/san-francisco-schools-transformed-power-meditation-n276301.

BREATHWORK

Getting in touch with your breath is a way to relax that requires no money and very little time. Therapists, body workers, yoga instructors, and healers of all kinds have used this ancient modality to reduce anxiety and relax the body and mind.

Incorporating breathwork into daily life is not difficult once the commitment to give it a go is made. To begin, set aside two to three minutes every day to recognize your breathing patterns. It helps me to put one hand on my belly and the other on my heart. That way I can feel and observe the breath coming in and out of my body. Go ahead and try it right now—one hand on the chest and the other on the belly. Close your eyes. Now breathe in and out, inflating and deflating your belly. Pay attention to it. When you grow antsy or start to think about the grocery list, go back to the breath. You see, when the breath gives you something to focus on, all those other worries have to take a back seat. Brilliant!

Many times throughout the day, I catch myself running hither and yon, and I feel as if I've been holding my breath the entire time. When I stop what I'm doing and focus on my breath, the in-and-out of it, I feel more "in my body" and less frantic within a minute or two. Breathwork can be your saving grace when you need to relax, especially if you are unable to do something more physical or have only a few minutes to spare.

CHIROPRACTIC ADJUSTMENTS

Chiropractic is a healing modality that extensively studies and explores the nervous system, which controls the sympathetic and parasympathetic conditions. Releasing stored stress through the manipulation of joints, especially the spinal column, is extremely effective in attaining a parasympathetic state.

Many of us plod through our daily lives unaware that we are stressed. Sometimes we feel it and call it accurately "that pain in the neck" or "that pain in my lower back." A misalignment in the joints or bones is called a subluxation, and chiropractors correct this with an adjustment. The "crack" you hear is the release of stored energy. I often land on my chiropractor's table in full sympathetic mode. After the session, I feel calm and grounded.

Chronic pain makes it difficult to achieve a parasympathetic state. Recent findings from a Washington State University study reported nearly one in five adults in America live with chronic pain, and the rates are even higher for women, seniors, and those who are obese.[4] Pain does not have to be permanent because the body has the innate ability to heal itself. Chiropractic treatment can aid the body in doing just that.

4. Katherine Roethel, "Chronic pain a hurdle for many, especially women, senior, obese," *San Francisco Chronicle*, November 12, 2014, accessed January 6, 2016, http://www.sfgate.com/health/article/Chronic-pain-a-hurdle-for-many-especially-women-5882325.php.

I would like to share a story with you regarding pain and the body's ability to heal. It's about a patient of mine who was fed up with taking the pain pills his primary care doctor told him he would have to continue for life. A work accident had left him with chronic pain from a broken pelvis and femur thirteen years prior. When we met, he was 38, overweight, smoking a pack of cigarettes a day, in despair, and had been addicted to painkillers for ten years. He had been given no alternatives to medication by his doctor and desperately wanted help. He wasn't going to take run-of-the-mill medical advice any more, and his wife was tired of seeing her husband "dumbed down by pain meds."

We developed a wellness plan that relied heavily on parasympathetic activities. It looked something like this:

- diet changed to vegetables, lean proteins, and healthy fats,

- significantly increased hydration that included two nutritional IVs a month for four months,

- supplements to address the chronic inflammation and buffer the pain receptors as he decreased the medication,

- increased para activities such as bike riding, walking, and building kit cars with his son,

- going to bed by 11 p.m. during the week,

- *weekly* chiropractic visits, and

- a new MD who believed in this patient's ability to decrease medications and was willing to work with us as a team.

Within five months, our patient was taking only 20 percent of his original pain medication, had lost 25 pounds, was biking 20 plus miles a week, and his quality of life was blossoming. He prioritized and made ample time for relaxation. With the help of his team, *he* was in charge, not his meds! Although he continues to smoke cigarettes on the weekends, he still hopes to quit one day. I keep reminding him: "One step at a time."

ORGASM

It would be a terrible oversight not to mention orgasm when discussing the parasympathetic nervous system. The majority of foreplay and the act of sex are actually stimulating and sympathetic. Yet, in order to achieve orgasm, the body and mind must reach a tipping point of feeling safe and relaxed. This point is what we call an orgasm, and it is para. I advocate for plenty of loving, pleasurable orgasms in your get para wellness plan.

VACATIONING

One of my tried-and-true ways of getting para is to take a vacation. This doesn't necessarily entail packing my suitcase and leaving on a jet plane. The term vacationing comes from vacate, as in vacating one's day-to-day routine. When I step out of my routine, my nervous system starts to release, my mind slows down, my creativity bubbles up, I sleep better, I smile more, and I clearly feel less muscle tension throughout my body. Sometimes it's as simple as driving to the beach or walking for a few hours in the woods with my dogs—most always without my phone.

NATURE

I read an article in *The New York Times* a few years back about how necessary it is for kids to have recess in school.[5] A study had concluded that eight and nine-year-olds behaved better in class if they had more than 15 minutes of recess per day. That, in my mind, is because they were allowed a para activity—and outside, not indoors. This same article referred to several studies with children, extolling the virtues of playtime and nature and the key roles each can play in learning, development, and general health.

Nature is a powerful healer, and I witnessed her healing forces firsthand while working at a wilderness therapy program for several years. Countless adolescents and young adults would arrive wired, tired, and often abusing drugs. They had very little connection to nature—or much of anything, actually. As the weeks passed, I saw these students reborn as they accepted nature's gifts. Some watched

---

5. Tara Parker-Pope, "The 3 R's? A Fourth Is Crucial, Too: Recess," *The New York Times*, Feb 23, 2009, accessed August 21, 2016, http://www.nytimes.com/2009/02/24/health/24well.html.

a full moon rise for the first time in their lives, and others were awestruck by the majesty of a thunderstorm as it tore across a valley. These moments in the wild, both subtle and fierce, demand attention and respect with little time for manipulation and argument. Time and time again, I observed with reverence as nature shifted these young people from loneliness and chaos to a place of humility and connection to self and others.

CHANGING THE MINDSET

Many of us are programmed to go-go-go from the time we stop taking naps in kindergarten. After school, children are shuttled from football practice to karate lessons or piano, rushed home to eat dinner, and then it's time to do homework. Not only are we a culture raised on sleep deprivation, we are also subjected to relaxing deprivation. By the time we are working adults, we are unaware of just how stressed we've become and choosing ways to relax doesn't even enter the picture. Engaging in a conversation with yourself or someone you trust about your stress level is a place to start. Ask yourself, how do you know when you are stressed and what do you do to counteract it? How does it feel to relax? Can you sit outside and watch the sunset without fidgeting? Can you be in the moment—enter the parasympathetic state? Awareness is the precursor to change.

Perhaps you are the "I have to see it to believe it type" who needs concrete evidence that you are stressed. This can be obtained by conducting a saliva test that will reveal your cortisol curve or lack of it. If your cortisol level is significantly high throughout the day, that's proof that you are stressed. If this is the case, and it almost always is, work with your licensed healthcare professional to add relaxation, supplementation, and real food to your lifestyle.

COMMUNITY

Many para activities can be solitary, but I believe some of the most powerful para times are shared. Watching a sunset in Big Sur with friends, sharing a homemade, locally grown dinner, or attending my book club can reset my para button. Back in 2000, I said the Serenity Prayer while holding hands with 55,000 people, and wow, was that a para moment!

God grant me the serenity to accept the things
I cannot change, the courage to change the things I can,
and the wisdom to know the difference.

We are all in this game of life together. Sometimes it takes community to allow us to feel safe and protected from the saber tooth tiger and the stresses of the world. *Rutgers Today* recently had an interesting article on the health effects of knowing we are all connected.[6] This article reiterated the importance of connection and community. The

---

6. Beth Salamon, "Rutgers Study Finds that Neighbors Improve Well-being in Middle and Later Life," *Rutgers Today*, September 17, 2014, accessed April 2, 2015, http://news.rutgers.edu/news/rutgers-study-finds-neighbors-improve-well-being-middle-and-later-life/20140916#.V7oEkZMrKRt.

research is clear that neighbors might not prevent us from feeling depressed, but they do contribute to what makes life worth living. Perhaps we can all relax just a little bit more when we get to know our neighbors.

If you are keen on the idea of creating a village, become familiar with an organization called Village to Village Network (Vtvnetwork.org). This volunteer group works to establish and maintain villages in the United States, Australia, and the Netherlands. The purpose is to foster village life that is loving, nurturing, and enjoyable.

CHAPTER 10 HEALTH RESOLUTION

Go back a few pages and look at my list of suggested para activities. Do one or two of them sound completely relaxing and luxurious to you? Do they seem almost decadent? If not, think up a list of your own. What activities would make you purr like a kitten? Write them down:

_____

_____

_____

_____

_____

_____

Now create some time for at least one of these activities each week. Then, go and do it! Give yourself the para you and your body desire and deserve.

CHAPTER 11

Just Move It

Now that you are getting more "para," let's also focus on movement as a part of your personal Health Revolution. I prefer the word "movement" to "exercise," simply because the word "exercise" sounds like a chore to many, including me. I grew up with the exercise mantra, "Five times a week for 20 minutes is a must to be healthy." That never resonated with me and still doesn't today. "Movement," however, sounds like play...interesting, more pleasant, and enjoyable. Both "movement" and "exercise" can provide the same outcome—improved health and fitness.

There is ample research supporting the benefits of movement. Movement pumps oxygen into our cells enhancing cardiovascular function and energy level. It also improves sleep, lightens mood, increases libido, offers enjoyment, and in many cases helps us relax. I see patients able to get more para especially when they participate in movement in nature and not in a busy, urban environment. In nature, folks don't just "get into the zone," they also connect to something greater. A 2015 study conducted at Stanford University revealed that participants who walked in nature, as opposed to those who walked in the city, had increased cognitive function and decreased anxiety and worry.[1] It isn't always convenient for all of us, especially those who live in a city, to get out into nature on a daily basis, but if you can change your routine and walk in the park instead of beside a busy freeway, it may be the healthier choice.

Many of us have been raised on the idea that we must "work out" and stay "fit." Today's go-go lifestyles imply that we must train for a marathon or hit the gym every day in order to take care of ourselves. This is simply not true. Yes, you do need to get off the couch, and the trick to that is to seek out a form of movement that does not seem so effortful and joyless. Such activities do exist, and you'll know one when you find it because there'll be no nagging voice in your head negating it. There will be no "I really don't want to do this, but I have to because it's good for me." No thinking, "I have to run five miles today, so no time to relax with my sweetie." No "I just burned 250 calories, so I can have two glasses of wine." That's the kind of mind chatter that truly won't benefit you over time. Let go of it,

1. Gregory N. Bratman, Gretchen C. Daily, Benjamin J. Levy, James J. Gross, "The Benefits of Nature Experience: Improved Affect and Cognition," Research Paper Stanford University, Science Direct, Landscape and Urban Planning, Volume 138, June 2015, 41-50, accessed June 12, 2016, doi March 2015, www.sciencedirect.com.

and find more favorable forms of movement that comple-
ment who you are and where you are in life.

TAKE THE FIRST STEP

An excellent movement to try out first is walking. It's
something most of us can do from the time we are twelve
months old until gravity and advanced age change all that.
Walking is a way to meet people, sincerely connect with
the environment, and free the mind. No power walks are
necessary. Get out there and amble at a pace that works
for you. Observe where the sun rises or sets, listen to your
breath, walk a dog, or stroll hand in hand with a loved one.
And oh, yes, stop and smell the roses—olfactory para. Try
walking once a week to a destination you would usually
drive a car, and notice how you experience the world differently. While living in a more urban environment, my walking has increased dramatically, and I feel more in touch
with local businesses, neighbors, and my neighborhood. A
fitness app on my smart phone tracks my mileage. I average
about 14 miles a week by walking with our dogs. And this
doesn't count my necessary-for-me hikes in the mountains
and on the beach.

If walking is not your idea of fun, then consider something you may not have ever considered before, such as a
martial arts class. They're a wonderful blend of East meets
West, with meditative qualities as well as physical benefits.
For example, tai chi and akido provide plenty of movement
but also focus on harmony within the body, which helps us

resist outside stresses. An overall theme of martial arts is to relax the body and quiet the mind, accessing an internal source of power both physical and mental. Given the many different styles of martial arts available, observe or check in with the teacher before arriving for a class. Once I made the mistake of signing up for a chi gong class only to find myself in a jujutsu class. Believe me, the two are not the same!

Movement in the form of dance comes in all shapes and sizes: ballet, line, ballroom, ecstatic, Soul Motion™, belly, hip-hop, swing, and pole dancing, which has caused quite a stir lately. The bottom line is that there are many ways to shake your booty. If classes aren't your cup of tea, then play your favorite album, and dance yourself around the house. Dance like you would if no one was watching you. Allow yourself to laugh and be silly.

> *ALLOW YOURSELF TO LAUGH AND BE SILLY.*

Biking is one of my favorite forms of movement. There is something about pedaling a bicycle that grounds me. Whether it's a leisurely ride to the store or a four-hour countryside tour, the rhythm of the bicycle settles my spirit. Biking has gained momentum with all age groups, so it's not difficult to find people nearby who would happily join you on a ride. Check out your local bike shop, and see what options are available. Then hop in the saddle, helmet on your head, and watch the world roll by.

Yoga is the Sanskrit word for union. Yoga uses breath, poses, and meditation to help you slow down enough to get para, while providing a variety of movements. There are many types of yoga: power, Hatha, yin, hot, and restorative, so give the different variations a try before deciding whether or not yoga is right for you. Too many of my patients have mistakenly thought they couldn't be injured in yoga class. Injuries, especially to shoulders, wrists, and knees, can happen. Move slowly, and let your teacher know about any previous injuries or limitations. Yoga is *your* movement. You do not have to keep up with anyone.

The type of movement that is most beneficial varies with a person's age, physical ability, and health status. To find the movement appropriate for you, tune into your physical and emotional capabilities, needs, and desires. I would not ask an elderly patient recovering from surgery to hop on a bike, though I might suggest a stretching class or water aerobics. If you know you're pushing the limits while doing something enjoyable, cautiously explore your unique, safe boundaries. If you're forcing yourself to do an activity because you feel you have to, I invite you to rethink this endeavor. Move so you enjoy it. Life is best when we look forward to something and relish the thought of doing it. That's what creates a desire to continue and gives us favorable memories.

Your form of movement can be unique. I have a patient who left banking after fifteen years and became a full-time farmer, because she discovered she was partial to the physical aspect of farming and the community of people involved.

The brave act of registering for a beginner's gardening class changed her life trajectory. She replaced a nine-to-five desk job that no longer fulfilled her with farming. That shift in movement was the beginning of her Health Revolution, and it all started when she took the time to notice she needed a change and then believed it was possible.

While you are discovering what movement nourishes you most, consider both solo and group activities. Some people like to move with only the company of their own thoughts and feelings. Others prefer movement to be a social event—a group bike ride followed by a healthy breakfast out, a tennis club tournament, or a guided nature hike. Try a little of each and see which form, solitary or social, you enjoy the most. Gift yourself the time to find the right movement for where you are in life today. Shake your booty, prune heirloom roses, glide across the snow on cross-country skis, or call "Fore!" on the golf course. Fill your heart with joy and your body with health, and if you so desire, do it all with people you love.

CHAPTER 11 HEALTH RESOLUTION

1. Write down all the different forms of movement you are interested in trying. Could you bicycle to work? Try a dance class? Join a rowing team? If you're stuck for ideas, ask someone whose lifestyle you admire what they do for movement.

_____

_____

_____

_____

_____

_____

_____

2. If you can't think of a type of movement that might be enjoyable, ponder what it is that's stopping you. Sometimes our resistance is an unwillingness to step out of a day-to-day routine and try something different. Are you not moving because you have a sore knee? Feel you are uncoordinated? Don't have time? All of those issues can be worked out with a trusted healthcare professional, mentor, or therapist. If you didn't have an issue standing in your way, what types of movement might you enjoy?

_____

_____

_____

_____

_____

_____

_____

3. Once you have a list of movements to consider, pick the top three. Find the time to try one, schedule it, and do it. If you love it, stick with it. If you don't, move on to number two.

CHAPTER 12
_____

A Healthy Community

Deepak Chopra, alternative medicine advocate, author, public speaker, and physician, insists we throw out the word "environment" and the idea that the environment or nature is something that exists outside of us. When I heard Dr. Chopra say this, I had one of those aha moments and thought, "I, too, want to inspire people to truly see themselves as part of nature and not separate from it." The two are profoundly connected—parts of the same, like the heart and brain are part of the human body—one living, breathing, complicated organism.

So many of us focus on cleaning up and saving the environment with little regard for cleaning up and saving ourselves, one person, one family, one community at a time. The state of our environment is a reflection of how all seven billion of us treat one another and ourselves. Pollution, deforestation, ozone depletion, mining, drilling, and fracking are all forms of destruction inflicted upon Earth and, consequently, upon humanity. *The Vis* comes from nature. If Earth is sick, we are sick.

There is a tipping point in healing. Whether a human is fighting for his life with an infection or planet Earth is working overtime to adjust air quality, there is a life force attempting to find balance. When we, as a civilization, cross the tipping point of no return, *The Vis* will no longer be able to bring humans or the Earth's ecosystems back to balance. Disease will win. Be that as it may, the forecast need not be so bleak. Ask yourself, "Am I moving one step closer to disease (ultimately death) or am I moving one step closer to health?" One by one, we can choose to respect and restore the environment beginning with assisting our own bodies. As this idea spreads from person to person, a mass healing will occur. This is The Health Revolution.

> *IF EARTH IS SICK,*
> *WE ARE SICK.*

Humankind has not woven the web of life.
We are but one thread within it.

Whatever we do to the web, we do to ourselves.

All things are bound together. All things connect.

—Chief Seattle, a Dkhw'Duw'Absh chief

THE SEARCH FOR OUR PEOPLE

Humans, generally speaking, like to be a part of something greater than their individual selves. For that reason, we seek community in many places: relationships, clubs, the Internet, religious affiliations, sports teams, schools, gyms, twelve-step meetings, coffee shops, service organizations, family, the military, universities, and places of employment. Communities offer each of us a sense of belonging, inspiration, challenge, purpose, and joy. In the same way we could do with more para in our lives, we also need communities that make our lives fuller, richer, easier, and healthier.

People tend to feel better when they are championed by and can relate to others. There is ample evidence that cancer and chronically ill patients backed by community support have better long-term outcomes than someone going it alone.[1] Surrounding oneself with people who reinforce well-thought-out decisions and who have hope for a positive outcome can only be beneficial. I have learned from my own life and from my practice that the person offering the assistance also benefits. You feel good. You have purpose. You are expressing love in a very palpable and practical way when you care for someone in need. If you have the opportunity to reach out and lend a helping hand to someone who is ill or experiencing a loss, go for it. Extending yourself in this way will have a positive effect on their mood and outlook, as well as your own.

1. "Coping with Cancer," accessed January 5, 2016, http://www.cancer.gov/cancertopics/coping/life-after-treatment/page 6.

COMMUNITY IN YOUR LIFE

When choosing community to enrich your life, make sure the group you are considering will fill that order. Community needs to jive with your philosophy, bolster you, and lovingly challenge you. Community should not make you feel anxious or bad about who you are. Sometimes you may feel trapped by a community you cannot easily change—your family or your workplace. In situations such as these, I recommend my patients seek professional help: a therapist, career counselor, or life coach. Find the right person to help you make positive change.

Take a moment to consider the communities you belong to now. Do these people inspire you? If not, consider a change. Perhaps you are not the same person you were when you joined the group months or years ago. Perhaps your spirit desires change and growth in ways that your current community simply can no longer offer. If so, depart with grace and gratitude for the service this group once provided. Then explore. Seek out new people who keep you on your toes—growing and living with great abundance.

THE WORKPLACE AS COMMUNITY

For many of us, the people with whom we work constitute an influential community. The word "company" derives from "commune" meaning to break bread with others. The question is, how and with whom do you choose to "break bread," both metaphorically as well as literally? What makes a workplace a healthy community? Does your company create community for employees? Do you create community for the company? Have you offered solutions and steered clear of complaining about what the CEO, managers, and directors should do for you and other employees? If not, perhaps it's time to bring your creativity and voice to the table. If it's not welcome, then search for another workplace or occupation where your voice will be regarded.

I once worked at a company consisting of the most eclectic group of people, and I often wondered what we had in common, how we "broke bread" together. I couldn't find a common denominator except for collecting a monthly paycheck. Aha! We weren't communing. We were just five individuals tackling tasks without a collaborative purpose. Additionally, there was little room for anyone to offer his or her creativity, and the CEO didn't believe in acknowledging people for their good work. In his words, "the paycheck was the acknowledgement." Needless to say, the energy felt stagnant, and I often heard, "It's only Wednesday, and I can't wait for Friday."

Life is too precious for this. In my experience, vibrant health and dynamic people do not flourish in stagnant environments, even when the paycheck sports an impressive sum. A toxic work environment lacks creativity and empowerment and breeds both physical and mental illness. When I worked at this company, I had to become honest with myself and accept that it was time to leave. Today, I am part of a dynamic movement burgeoning with the opportunity to express new ideas, creativity, fun, individuality, and collaboration. This is the type of work I am talking about: healthy people collectively building a place, a community, a revolution in which they can thrive.

I have been fortunate to attend workshops (another form of community) taught by Matthew and Terces Engelhart, authors, organic farmers, and founders and owners of Café Gratitude and Gracias Madre restaurants. Gracious teachers to thousands, they have deliberately created healthier work environments by educating others about clear communication and intentions. One great example of this is to refrain from all forms of gossiping. The purpose is to create a safe workplace that fosters freedom of expression for everyone. Gossip provokes anxiety and worry in people that can lead to depression, insomnia, high blood pressure, headaches, substance abuse, and many other health ailments. How much gossip happens where you work and spend many hours each day? Are you a contributor or a target of this hurtful practice? Perhaps it's time to effect change and create a no-gossip, less stressful work environment.

TAKE YOUR PICK

Besides work, you can find community just about everywhere. We naturally seek out others who have similar interests and goals. America is still the land of diversity, so take your pick and dive in. Clubs, neighborhood committees, recreation centers, YMCAs, and other public facilities are affordable ways to meet people. Spiritual communities such as churches and temples, Zen centers, ashrams, and retreat centers are other great places to explore.

If you desire an outlet for your art, seek a community that fosters creativity, a loving place to work, and maybe even an occasional potluck dinner. If you want to start a business, you might join an entrepreneur group to learn the ins and outs of a business start-up. Perhaps a meditation group can help you manage the stress of starting such a business.

Of course, family and friends make up our most immediate and intimate community. If we are fortunate, they accompany us throughout the joys and sorrows of our lives. Seth Godin, author, blogger, and one of my mentors, talks about each of us being the sum of the five people with whom we surround ourselves the most, whether they are co-workers, teachers, a spouse, friends, family, or neighbors. Currently, who are the five most pronounced influencers in your life?

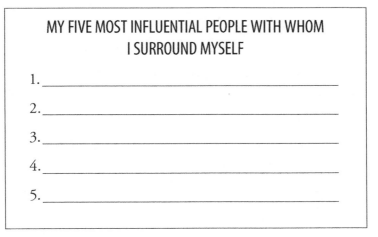

MY FIVE MOST INFLUENTIAL PEOPLE WITH WHOM I SURROUND MYSELF

1. _____

2. _____

3. _____

4. _____

5. _____

As adults, we all have choice in this matter. Do the individuals you listed add richness and depth to your life? If they are not influencing you in a positive way, perhaps it's time to consider slowly or quickly backing out of some of these relationships. Also, ask yourself, "Are you contributing to their fulfillment, and as a result, building a strong healthy community together?"

If your list fills you with gratitude, acknowledge these people for the gift that they are. Take them to lunch, send a letter, or hug them and let them know how much they matter. Simple acknowledgment and appreciation can make someone's day, and very importantly, help build trusting and lasting relationships.

BREAKING BREAD FOR REAL

Dining with family and friends is one of the most beautiful and rewarding expressions of community. It's a place to feed the mind, the heart, the soul…and the belly.

As a teenager, I had the opportunity to visit Europe a few times with family and friends. I have vivid memories of folks sitting for hours around tables filled with fruit, bread, cheese, wine, and conversation punctuated with laughter. I asked my grandmother during one trip, "What do they talk about for all that time?"

She remarked, "Everything, my sweets. Food, art, politics, jokes, family, dreams."

I had not experienced anything like that back home in America. Most of the time my family ate in front of the TV with not much conversation. Prior to my stay in Europe I thought that everyone ate mindlessly, that dining wasn't anything special. In Europe, I didn't see anyone walking around with a coffee-to-go or a *panini* wrapped in foil. For Europeans, food was (and in some cases still is) more than gobbling up the meals placed before us; it is a time to be together, to be thoughtful, and grateful.

When ideas, connection, and love are spread around the table, life can carry on in a more meaningful, honest, and deeply felt way. The right community at the table, at work, at the food shelter where you volunteer, can and will contribute to your overall health and wellness.

I invite you to view your community(ies) as an extension of your mental, emotional, spiritual, and physical health. Community building is a way you can actively take part in The Health Revolution.

CHAPTER 12 HEALTH RESOLUTION

Have you been toying with the idea of taking a class, joining a club, or reaching out to a side of the family with whom you've lost contact? Then I urge you to take an action step. Write down five communities you are interested in:

1. _____

2. _____

3. _____

4. _____

5. _____

Now, join one of these communities this week. You will be welcomed.

CHAPTER 13

Disease Du Jour

In the early chapters of this book, the naturopathic concept of *vis mediatrix naturae*, the healing power of nature, was introduced. There is another naturopathic belief that accompanies *vis mediatrix naturae*, which is that disease is a process caused by an imbalance in the body's natural homeostasis. The naturopathic doctor believes that disease can be abated and very often eliminated by restoring health to the entire body. In contrast, standard Western medicine assumes that most disease is an entity that can be eliminated or suppressed with medication, and in some cases, surgery.

Despite great efforts to combat disease with standard medicine, it is rampant in America. Disease costs money, time, energy, and lives. Cancer alone affects over

1.5 million Americans a year,[1] heart disease over 25 million,[2] and diabetes 29 million.[3]

We, the people, are becoming increasingly ill. Then we search in all the wrong places to rid ourselves of these ailments by popping a magic pill!

WHAT'S SO DIFFERENT ABOUT TODAY?

Patients sometimes ask me why we are so sick and stressed in this time of "medical advancement." I can say with no hesitation that chronic disease is more prevalent today because of

- food grown in depleted soil and then heavily processed,

- lack of movement of the body,

- not enough sunlight or time in nature,

- living in a polluted environment,

- suppression of symptoms via medications, and

1. "Cancer Facts & Figures 2014," accessed January 18, 2016, http://www.cancer.org/acs/groups/content/@research/documents/webcontent/acspc-042151.pdf.

2. "Fast Stats, Heart Disease," Centers for Disease Control and Prevention, accessed January 18, 2016, http://www.cdc.gov/nchs/fastats/heart-disease.htm.

3. "Diabetes Home," Centers for Disease Control and Prevention, accessed January 18, 2016, http://www.cdc.gov/diabetes/data/statistics/2014statisticsreport.html.

- a medical system that minimizes the importance of patient empowerment and education regarding positive lifestyle changes.

It may be argued that the increase in chronic disease in our modern time is due to longer life spans, but that does not explain the rise in childhood diabetes, asthma, heart disease, and obesity. As a nation, even our children are becoming sicker and sicker. Perhaps more than ever, it's time to question and demand change in the engrained systems that hurt us: how we grow and prepare food, how we take care of the Earth, and how we go about dealing with our health. Let's put our money and faith into the hands of local organic farmers and doctors who listen—those who are part of The Health Revolution Solution.

The Health Revolution is all about preventing illness, but it is also about providing compassionate and affordable care for those who are ill and in need. Education is the first step to understanding what is going on with us as individuals and as a species. So let's take a look at a few diseases that are on the rise, prevalent, and often curable. Yes, *curable*, meaning that a person diagnosed with a given disease may be restored to health.

DIGESTIVE PROBLEMS:
TREAT THE GUT. TREAT THE GUT. TREAT THE GUT.

Our guts are in distress. They cry out in the form of disease such as irritable bowel syndrome (IBS), inflammatory bowel disease (IBD), Crohn's disease, Celiac disease, bloating, SIBO (small intestinal bacterial overgrowth), gastritis, burping, GERD (gastro esophageal reflux disease), H. Pylori infection, ulcers, stomach and colon cancer, diarrhea, constipation, gluten intolerance, food sensitivities, and food allergies.

What the heck is causing this major disruption of our digestive systems?

There are four main culprits: 1) lack of nutrient-dense food, 2) GMOs, 3) the depleted quality of soil that food is grown in, and 4) increased stress coupled with our go-go lifestyles, which leads to an inability to digest food properly.

When humans were literally running from the saber tooth tiger, they weren't simultaneously gulping a protein shake. Today, we drive and eat, work and eat, watch horrific sensational news and eat—all of which makes for a population with digestive issues. When we are unable to calmly digest food, the stress hormone, cortisol, is stimulated. Too much cortisol impedes digestion enzymes from doing their job and the absorption of nutrients. Our bodies become depleted of fuel (nutrients) and our cells starve. Eventually this leads to disease. We must be able to obtain nutrients from the food we eat, or else we are in big trouble.

Discovering the underlying cause and patiently taking the time necessary to heal can resolve most digestive problems. Work with a knowledgeable, licensed healthcare professional in your area. What's impeding your digestive system? Is it a food sensitivity, infection, diminished digestion enzymes, poor eating habits, or a combination of them all?

The undeniable truth, however, is this: favorable gut health is reliant upon eating real, organic, and local food and taking the time to relax and enjoy it.

FOOD SENSITIVITIES

In 1996, when I had that severe negative reaction to the extraction of my wisdom teeth, I felt and looked like Frankenstein's monster. The well-intentioned nurse at the dental office said, "Oh honey, just take some aspirin. Tomorrow it will be all better." But somehow I didn't think so. I felt deep inside of me that there had to be another way to deal with severe mouth and neck pain, headache, and fear.

A week later, I had my first and only anaphylactic reaction to a seasonal allergy shot. I had been receiving the same injection since high school with no ill effects. I knew intuitively that the removal of my wisdom teeth and my anaphylactic reaction were connected, and that something was terribly wrong with my body—something that wasn't going to be fixed by an aspirin, a new allergy medication, or my same old doctors.

In search of a better answer, I visited a recommended chiropractor. She gave me a gentle but effective spinal adjustment that reset my nervous system. I was able to exit the "fight or flight" state I was in and relax. I could turn my neck without pain. I could breathe deeply once again. But, just as importantly, this doctor listened to my tale of woe, and after I answered a few direct questions, suggested I stop eating all gluten and soy for 30 days. She suspected these substances were part of what my body was reacting against so violently. She was pretty certain I had a food sensitivity. I asked her which foods contained gluten and she replied, "Gluten is in everything you are eating: cereal, pizza, pasta, beer, cookies, pastries, bagels..." She was right. At that time in my life, my whole diet was gluten based, with a little bit of soy in the form of a popular energy bar. I cried all the way home, adding severely swollen eyes to my list of maladies. What the hell would I eat?

That visit to the chiropractor was the catalyst to my gluten-free days. And trust me, going gluten-free in 1996 was much harder than it is today. Nowadays, just about anything in a gluten-free form is easy to find in stores and restaurants. (Remember to stick to real food and not processed gimmicks.) Within weeks of eliminating gluten from my diet, many of my symptoms faded to memory. Do I have Celiac disease? No. Do I become sick when I eat gluten? Yes, and I have ended up in the hospital twice from acute GI distress and dehydration as a result of trying to re-introduce gluten into my diet. Not fun and expensive, too! It turns out soy isn't a major problem for me, though soy milk can lead to bloating and discomfort. While researching soy, however, I discovered that it is used as a filler in numerous packaged foods, so I gathered valuable awareness in the process.

Looking back, I realize that my body had been reacting for some time to the overload of gluten I was consuming, and simply said "enough" when I topped it all off with an allergy shot and medications for a wisdom tooth extraction. My immune system, which is also in the gut, was tired of working overtime to fend off gluten and offered me a big wake-up call. I wish I had listened to my body earlier. Years of dealing with a bloated belly, low energy, unexplained rashes and hives, sneezing, mood swings, and cravings for more and more gluten could have been avoided.

I find an increasing number of patients are becoming sensitive to foods. Perhaps this is due to preservatives, chemicals, and GMOs in our food. Perhaps it's the rushing around we engage in while we are eating and drinking. Whatever the reason, it's undeniable that our bodies are telling us something. But who is listening?

Sensitivities are not the same as food allergies. I am not referring to an anaphylactic reaction to food. I'm talking about little health quirks and irritations that add up to just not feeling well.

If you are experiencing symptoms and don't readily have an explanation for them, perhaps your body is telling you that something you're eating is not agreeable to your digestive system. Many people go years, or even a lifetime, not knowing they have food sensitivities. I encounter too many patients who have been taking over-the-counter

SYMPTOMS THAT MAY INDICATE FOOD SENSITIVITY

Joint pain	Headache
Racing heart	Allergies
Stuffy sinuses	Sinus infections
Chronic infections	Nausea
Bloating	Skin rashes
Digestive issues	PMS
Lack of libido	Brain fog
Fatigue	Depression
Anxiety/panic attacks	Sleep issues

antihistamines for five to 20 years and never once considered their allergy symptoms could be related to the food they consume and not the external environment. Heal the gut, which strengthens the immune system, and most people can minimize and eliminate the need for over-the-counter antihistamines.

If you have a food sensitivity, your body produces antibodies as a reaction to the disagreeable food. You can determine which food is causing the issue by 1) obtaining a blood test, or 2) doing an elimination diet.

ELIMINATION DIETS

Discerning food sensitivities is not always easy and takes diligence. To do so, you need to eliminate a suspect food from your diet entirely, as I did in 1996 with gluten and soy. Willingness, interest, and curiosity about your body (usually spurred by a chronic health condition) make the process less of a chore and more of an adventure. Keeping track of what you eat and the resultant symptoms in a food diary is a great way to narrow down which foods may be causing discomfort.

Here is a list of foods that I find patients are most sensitive to:

COMMON FOOD SENSITIVITY CULPRITS

Corn	Soy	Nuts and Peanuts
Dairy	Alcohol	Eggs
Sugar	Yeast	Gluten (wheat, rye, barley, couscous, spelt)

To learn how to detect a food sensitivity, let's take a hypothetical case. You've noticed for the last six months that something is upsetting your stomach and you keep getting colds that grow into sinus infections. You discuss this with friends (or better yet, an integrative physician) and suspect dairy may be the cause of these symptoms. To know with more certainty, you cease eating dairy for 14 days. And yes, this is no easy task, but to carry out a reliable test you need to be strict with yourself for this amount of time. Sometimes, it's extremely helpful to find a partner who will follow the same protocol. Misery, or as I like to say in this case "discovery," loves company. If you are eating prepared or processed foods, be sure to read the labels. Dairy, gluten, soy, and some form of sugar are thrown into almost everything that's packaged.

On day 15, reintroduce dairy. Refrain from adding any other new food types into your diet, so you can make sure you are monitoring the reintroduction of dairy only. Consume dairy with every meal: cheese in your scrambled eggs and cream in your coffee at breakfast, cottage cheese atop your salad for lunch, and perhaps a little ice cream in the evening, after a baked potato with sour cream. Over the next few minutes up to 48 hours, be attentive to how your body responds. Do you notice any of the old symptoms returning—too much phlegm, a stomachache, or a stuffy nose? If so, you can be pretty certain that your body is sensitive to dairy.

Another example: You suspect corn isn't agreeing with you, causing stomach pain, bloating, and diarrhea. You don't eat it for 14 days, reintroduce it on day 15 and notice no side effects. Great, then your body isn't reacting negatively to corn in the same way mine wasn't sensitive to soy. But don't stop there! Investigate further. Could gluten be the issue? If so, the next step is to cut out wheat, rye—all the grains and foods that contain gluten.

It's essential to reintroduce one food item at a time. I often see patients, friends, and family who are trying to pinpoint a food sensitivity go on a cleanse eliminating many types of food, and when the cleansing period is over, they make the huge mistake I call "turbo reintroduction." They eat a cheeseburger and shake (gluten, dairy, and sugar) or cheese tamales (dairy and corn) and feel horrible. Not only do they feel terrible, but they also do not know which food has caused the undesirable symptoms. If you've been on a cleanse eliminating several types of food, allow 24 to 48 hours between reintroducing each food, one at a time.

Once the food sensitivity is identified, the real fun begins: that of healing your gut over time. Begin by eliminating the food entirely for three to six months, all the while supporting your gut and immune system with a healthful diet, foods that promote excellent digestion such as fermented foods, recommended supplements, and, of course, lifestyle changes geared to decreasing stress. When you feel great and are asymptomatic, you can reintroduce the food(s) one at a time and see how your body reacts. You may be pleasantly surprised to learn that you can eat the culprit food once again in moderation.

INFLAMMATION

There are two different classifications for inflammation: acute and chronic. Acute inflammation exists when there has been trauma to bodily tissue. Think about the redness and soreness of a swollen, twisted ankle. These symptoms are the result of increased blood flow and neutrophils being sent to the affected area to aid in healing. This is the

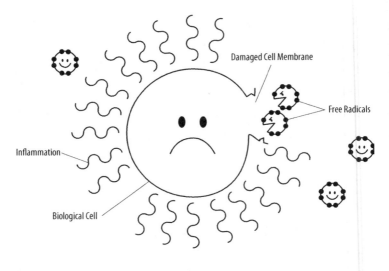

Damaging Free Radicals

body's natural and healthy response to repair the injury. Acute inflammation is finite and usually lasts for a short period of time.

Chronic inflammation is prolonged and doesn't heal, but damages bodily tissue. Practically every disease process is linked to chronic inflammation. Diseases with names that end in "itis" are inflammatory processes: arthritis (joints), colitis (inflammation of the colon), cystitis (the bladder), dermatitis (the skin), and thyroiditis (the thyroid). Chronic inflammation is partly caused by environmental factors such as pesticides, fungicides, and herbicides in our food supply and pollutants in our water, soil, and air. It is also part of aging. All of these events cause free radicals to form in the body.

Free radicals are an atom or a group of atoms with one unpaired electron in their makeup, which means that the atom(s) are unstable and not part of a healthy body. When the body attempts to eliminate free radicals, inflammation is the result. Unchecked, free radicals wreak havoc on cellular structures, initiating a cascade of pro-inflammatory genetic signals that ultimately result in cell death or worse, uncontrolled cell growth, the hallmark of cancer.

I help many patients develop wellness plans that address chronic inflammation. They often come to me complaining of the following symptoms:

SYMPTOMS INDICATING CHRONIC INFLAMMATION

Sore and achy joints

Swollen ankles

Headaches

Digestion problems, diarrhea and/or constipation

Blood sugar ups and downs

Difficulty sleeping

Bouts of depression

Allergies

Increased menstrual cramping

Bleeding gums while flossing or brushing

Cancer

Diet is the place to start when dealing with inflammation. Cut back on eating processed foods and add nutrient-dense, real food to your diet. Load up on vegetables and fruits, many of which (berries in particular) are anti-inflammatories and antioxidants. Antioxidants stop the cell damage caused by free radicals, also known as oxidants. Supplemental antioxidants, such as NAC (N-acetyl cysteine, a modified form of the amino acid Cysteine), vitamin C, vitamin E, R-Lipoic acid, turmeric, and green tea are definitely warranted. Water, lots of it, pooping daily, and a weekly sauna will help expel the free radicals as well.

Chronic inflammation, because it is relentless, wears down the body. It can also wear down the spirit. I highly recommend you seek a licensed healthcare practitioner who will listen to your whole story and devise a wellness plan that addresses your whole person. Tamping out the prolonged burn of chronic inflammation can be a long road. My desire is for you to have a trusted healthcare advisor during the entire process.

CHRONIC ACHES AND PAINS

Pain disrupts our quality of life. It's difficult to work, play, and remain optimistic when you hurt all the time. Headaches, neck and back pain, joint pain, pre-menstrual cramps, and pain from injuries, as well as from chemotherapy and radiation, send a lot of folks into the doctor's office looking for relief. Most often the remedy suggested is in the form of medication.

There is no shortage of pain medication available over the counter and by prescription. Doctors and patients, as a team, often strive to find the sweet spot that allows for pain relief without creating a dependency. The over-prescription of pain medications has become such a problem that many states have enacted laws requiring patients to visit their doctor every three months for refills. Still, patients are often over-medicated and out of touch with their pain. This is regrettable because pain is the first clue to learning what is occurring in the body. Pain is the body screaming for help. It's an alarm that something is not right, a sign of stagnancy, inflammation, and degeneration. To treat pain, the first thing to ask is, "What is my pain trying to tell me?"

WHAT IS MY PAIN TRYING TO TELL ME?

When I discuss pain with patients, I ask them a multitude of questions: Where is it exactly? When did it start? What does it feel like? What does it prevent you from doing? My approach is to discover what's causing the pain, remediate the cause, and gradually decrease medication with the assistance of the prescribing doctor until medication is no longer needed. It is important to find a doctor who will support the goal of eventually discontinuing medication.

All pain is not equal in intensity. Every patient has a different story and a different way of expressing it. The most effective and compassionate treatment is geared toward the individual patient's story and not to a generalized idea of pain. Physical, emotional, and mental states must all be discussed and addressed. For example, anxiety is often associated with chronic pain. I had a patient in his twenties who came to me with chronic knee and hip pain, the result of high school football and basketball injuries. Over a period of three years, he had become dependent on narcotics, taking them before his physical workouts, which were important to him. He had become so anxious about the pain he would have to endure that narcotics became a solution. It was sometimes difficult for him to distinguish which was worse—the pain or the anxiety of the anticipated pain.

As his doctor, I began by listening to this young man's story. I heard him and acknowledged both his anxiety and his pain. Together, we developed a wellness plan targeting the inflammation that was the underlying cause of his pain. Over a period of four months, we bolstered his immune system with anti-inflammatory foods and supplements, regulated his blood sugar by adding healthy fats to his diet and cutting back on alcohol, and purchased alternate workout shoes that offered better support.

As for anxiety management, I suggested he see a family therapist. I suspected some of his anxiety and pain were related to his father abruptly passing away while my patient was a star athlete in high school. Therapy helped him see the relationship between his father's death and his own pain. The combination of my guidance and the support of a therapist gave this patient enough strength to eliminate the narcotics from his life without addiction counseling. Addressing this man's health, both physical and emotional, gave him the foundation he needed to establish a life free of narcotics.

Pain is a bully, making a person feel cornered with no place to go for help. But pain can be reduced and often eliminated when the patient (and the doctor) learns to trust and collaborate with the body's innate ability to heal itself.

ELEVATED CHOLESTEROL

Elevated cholesterol is a condition found in all types of people—skinny, athletic, young, elderly, vegetarian, and vegan included. An abundance of cholesterol can create plaque or fatty deposits within arteries, inhibiting or blocking blood flow. This can lead to clots, strokes, heart attack, and chronic inflammatory issues. Post-menopausal women often develop elevated cholesterol due to the relationship between hormones and cholesterol. The bottom line is that cholesterol-lowering medications, called statins, are overprescribed in America with no discussion of ever getting off of them. Statins have known side effects including liver inflammation, muscle fatigue, and muscle atrophy. Between 2011 and 2012, more than one-quarter (27.9 percent) of adults aged 40 and older reported using a prescription cholesterol-lowering medication in the past 30 days. This was an increase from 2003 to 2004, when one in five adults (19.9 percent) used a cholesterol-lowering medication.[4]

If your cholesterol is high, the questions to ask yourself and your physician are: "Why is my cholesterol high?" "What is my good (HDL) to bad cholesterol (LDL) ratio?" "Can I lower my cholesterol without taking medication?"

My answer to the last question for most patients is "yes." If you are willing to make diet and lifestyle changes, then chances are you can avoid taking a statin. Find an integrative doctor who will help you lower cholesterol naturally.

By now, it's pretty clear that there is no one-size-fits-all treatment plan for patients in the eyes of a naturopathic doctor. However, for my patients with elevated cholesterol, diet and family history are immediate topics of conversation. Understanding genetic predisposition and adjusting diet and body movement routines are the first line of action. To help the body through this transition, there are botanical herbs, supplements, and foods that help lower the bad cholesterol while increasing the good cholesterol. These include niacin (vitamin B3), fish oil, fresh garlic, green tea, and soluble fibers such as beans, apples, lentils, and carrots.

4. Qiuping Gu, M.D., Ph.D.; Ryne Paulose-Ram, Ph.D., M.A.; Vicki L. Burt, Sc.M., R.N.; and Brian K. Kit, M.D., M.P.H., "Prescription Cholesterol-lowering Medication Use in Adults Aged 40 and Over: United States, 2003-2012," CDC Publications and Information Products, NCHS Data Brief No. 177, December 2014, accessed February 13, 2016, http://www.cdc.gov/nchs/data/databriefs/db177.htm.

This protocol may seem simple, but it is effective. I haven't kept strict statistics, but close to 90 percent of the patients I have worked with in this fashion have been able to discontinue cholesterol medications and live a healthier, more empowered life.

OBESITY

There are many synonyms that can soften or heighten the effect of the word "obese"—fat, chunky, *zaftig*, big, overweight, and plus-sized to name a few. No matter what you label it, the hard, cold truth is that obesity is a disease and an epidemic in America. Worse yet, additional medical issues such as joint pain, high cholesterol, heart disease, and diabetes often accompany obesity.

In 2012, the Robert Wood Johnson Foundation reported that over 50 percent of Americans will be obese by the year 2030.[5] This figure ensures a steady revenue stream for the Western medical model. The F (food) part of the FDA ensures that there are plenty of nutrient-deprived processed foods, sugars, preservatives, and GMOs to eat, and the D (drug) part provides medications for the diseases very likely caused by the foods! It's a perfect feedback loop to generate revenue for hospitals, insurance providers, and pharmaceutical companies at the cost of American health. And yet,

5. "F as in Fat: How Obesity Threatens America's Future in 2013," Trust for America's Health and Robert Wood Johnson Foundation, September 2012, accessed August 21, 2016, http://healthyamericans.org/report/108/.

we need to take responsibility, too. We are literally eating ourselves into the grave.

The Skinny on Obesity is a seven-part documentary series produced by University of California Television that is truly worth watching on YouTube. The first episode

WE ARE LITERALLY EATING OURSELVES INTO THE GRAVE.

alone, *The Skinny on Obesity: An Epidemic for Every Body,*[6] is an eye opener. This video explains how and why obesity, which has had a 40 percent increase over the past 30 years, is an American public health problem—one that impacts us all and should no longer be ignored.

Curing obesity involves much more than eating less food and exercising more. It's more than responding to a slick, celebrity-endorsed weight loss plan seen on TV. It's about learning the importance of eating nutrient-dense foods and fewer processed foods, understanding genetic hurdles in your family, managing stress in your life, and finding a community that supports you and your healthier lifestyle.

6. "The Skinny on Obesity: An epidemic for Every Body" with Dr. Lustig, UCSF Mini Medical School for the Public [Health and Medicine] [Show ID: 16717], Uploaded on July 30, 2009, http://www.uctv.tv/shows/ The-Skinny-on-Obesity-Ep-1-An-Epidemic-for-Every-Body-23305.

TYPE 2 DIABETES

Type 2 diabetes is truly an unnecessary epidemic. The processed food industry participates as the movie director, while American consumers act out the horror show: eating, becoming sick with diabetes, going on medication, never getting to the root of the problem, and eventually dying. It's time for the curtain to come down on this type of picture show!

Type 2 diabetes occurs when the body is unable to effectively manage glucose (often derived from carbohydrates like soda, bread, cereal, alcohol, candy, and sugar) via insulin. The hormone insulin is responsible for the amount of glucose being transported from your bloodstream to your cells, where it is used as fuel. High concentrations of glucose remaining in the bloodstream translate into diabetes.

Diabetes in the American population is so prevalent that medical doctors have resorted to prescribing medications in order to prevent it. This translates into big money for pharmacology. Why else would you prescribe a medication even before the disease process starts? This type of healthcare is a win for Big Pharma and a loss for wellness.

In 1992, the president of the American Diabetes Association, Francine Ratner Kaufman, MD, stated that it was rare for most pediatric centers to have patients with type 2 diabetes. By 1994, type 2 diabetes accounted for up to 16 percent of new cases of pediatric diabetes in urban areas, and by 1999, it accounted for eight to 45 percent of new cases depending on geographic location.[7] We saw this epidemic coming, but what did we do as a country? We started prescribing medications to our youth, another band-aid approach to the much larger underlying cultural issue of feeding our kids junk food laden with sugar, carbohydrates, and GMOs. Furthermore, we chose not to emphasize, and in some cases ignore, the direct correlation between processed sugar and type 2 diabetes.

Kidney disease, often the result of long-term, uncontrolled diabetes, is also rampant in our culture, as evidenced by the proliferation of neighborhood dialysis centers often conveniently located across the street from numerous fast food establishments. If you ever have the occasion to visit a dialysis center, notice if they offer soda, juice, candy, or donuts to their clientele. Chances are they do, and each of these foods perpetuates the problem. It's similar to serving cocktails at an AA meeting.

Diseases such as type 2 diabetes are curable. Yes, it's true. In most cases, this disease is curable if the patient is willing to fully participate in his or her care, which includes diet change, body movement of some variety, supplementation, and most crucially, daily monitoring of the blood sugar level. The more blood sugar levels are understood and monitored, the more likely the patient can be cured of the disease.

7. American Diabetes Association, "Diabetes Journals" accessed July 20, 2015, http://clinical.diabetesjournals.org/content/20/4/217.full.

Traditionally, diabetes is treated with medications, labs every three months, and perhaps some "nutritional advice." This advice often consists of teaching diabetics to calculate their medication based on how many carbohydrates they consume, with little to no education about the role carbohydrates play in the reason why they are sick. Diabetics should not eat an abundance of carbohydrates, but if they do, especially at one sitting, there must be a balance of healthy fats and proteins to offset the effects.

I have a friend whose doctor says he's doing "great" managing his type 2 diabetes—even though he has poor eyesight, is morbidly obese, has had a leg amputated due to diabetic complications, and has numbness in his remaining foot. The "great" comment was based on his A1C lab result (the blood test used to monitor blood sugar levels), which remained mostly in the normal zone due to his medications. It breaks my heart that this man has chosen not to pursue care outside his insurance network. With alternative healthcare, I believe he would be free of type 2 diabetes in less than a year, or at a minimum, enjoying a higher standard of living. This is not uncommon—for folks to choose a medication over reclaiming health—especially when their doctor is supportive of that choice. Many people don't want to change their habits. They choose to remain in their comfort zone, eat too many carbohydrates, and take pills. And to be fair, some folks feel they cannot afford an integrative doctor because their insurance won't cover this type of care. The failure of insurance to cover alternative healthcare is a major reason The Health Revolution needs to be in full gear: Everyone should have access to affordable care with the practitioner of his or her choice.

Years ago, I had a gentleman come to me with several symptoms pointing to poorly managed diabetes, and his A1C lab result was 13 percent (very high). Within nine months of following my health guidelines, not only was his A1C in a safe zone of less than six percent, but he had also lost a significant amount of weight, was enjoying daily exercise, and had begun to sift through the loss of his father with whom he had been very close. He took a few supporting supplements throughout this process, and over time, with the guidance of his MD and myself, was able to stop all his medication. Fifteen years later, this wonderful, artistic man is still free of type 2 diabetes and living a healthy, fulfilling life with his wife.

CANCER

If we take a step back from focusing only on the cancer affecting humans and also acknowledge the cancer inflicted upon our planet, we can see how we must take a truly holistic approach to "fight" this disease. Cancer in humans is prevalent because our Earth is sick, and if our Earth is sick, then we are sick. Earth has stage four cancer, and we see metastatic signs all over her. Much of our soil is depleted, barren, diseased, and polluted. There's a hole burned in our atmosphere. The oceans are over-fished and littered with plastic ranging from tiny micro-pellets to suffocating bags. We are cutting, burning, paving, pumping, fracking, and mining our lands to death. Earth is sick, and the symptoms of drought, extreme weather, infertility, and pollution are the evidence.

Greed and carelessness are too often getting in the way of good health for us as individuals and for the planet we inhabit. Native American spirituality teaches that we are all One—animals, humans, plants, mountains—everything. If we are treating this planet badly, we are treating ourselves badly. We can build walls around our model green communities and turn off the bad news, but that doesn't stop the disease. We must come to accept the fact that we and the Earth are one, and that the time is definitely here to take action and heal us all.

Cancer is one of the leading causes of death worldwide.[8] I treat many patients with cancer. In my practice, I have seen an increase of lung cancer in non-smokers, brain cancer in otherwise thriving middle-aged men and women, and colon cancer occurring much earlier in life. There's no denying that there is abundant cancer research being conducted, but here is the problem: the focus is mostly on finding a *cure* for cancer. What about the *why* of cancer? Instead of spending billions of dollars on curing cancer with medication, how about putting at least some of these funds towards addressing the root causes? Let's clean up our food and water supplies by supporting organic farmers and provide pure food and drink that isn't delivered in plastic

8. "Cancer Statistics," National Cancer Institute, accessed May 25, 2016, www.cancer.gov.

containers or through lead pipes. Let's stop spewing toxins into the air. Let's study and learn about genetic risk factors. Let's train more integrative doctors, who will educate and guide us along the way and encourage alternative therapies in conjunction with chemotherapy and radiation. If we do all that, *The Vis* will be alive and well, and so will we.

When cancer is diagnosed, I urge patients to obtain two or three opinions, especially before starting treatment. UCLA Cancer Centers, MD Anderson Care Centers, Riordan Clinic in Wichita, Kansas, Oncology Association of Naturopathic Physicians, Cancer Center of America, and the Mayo Clinic are all highly reputable options to explore. Don't be afraid to interview prospective oncologists, radiologists, or naturopathic doctors and ask how many cancers just like yours they have treated. Ask about their success rates and *how they measure that success.* These are key questions that will help you assemble the best of the best for your treatment, as well as the most compassionate and collaborative care.

The world of oncology is advancing quickly in regard to genetic testing that can lead to more accurate medication choices and immunotherapy, which uses the immune system's natural ability to both detect and treat cancer.[9] This type of medical advancement, along with complementary treatments such as nutritional IVs, real food, proper supplementation, and emotional and moral support

---

9. "Immunotherapy: Using the Immune System to Treat Cancer," NIH National Cancer Institute, accessed February 13, 2016, http://www.cancer.gov/research/areas/treatment/immunotherapy-using-immune-system.

from your community, will reduce the side effects of chemotherapy and radiation, enhance quality of life, and promote healing.

DEPRESSION AND ANXIETY

Chances are that you or someone you know have experienced depression, anxiety, or both. Given that there is a major shortage of qualified mental health professionals available to us,[10] the problems with insurance reimbursement, and the fact that behavioral health issues are still considered somewhat taboo, it makes sense that many patients and physicians feel they have nowhere to turn except the prescription pad. As I write this, Kaiser Permanente mental health clinicians are picketing outside their Oakland, California, campus. Their grievance is that they are not allocated enough time or money to fulfill the needs of patients. Many insurance companies pay for only six to eight visits to a psychologist or therapist yearly, which is barely enough time to get started. Additionally, they refuse to pay for in-patient treatment longer than a 72-hour safety hold for individuals dealing with depression or anxiety. Once again, we see the "time dilemma" rearing its ugly head in the world of medicine. Wouldn't it be nice if our current medical system effectively supported people with mental health concerns and offered them opportunities

10. Melissa Dahl, "There's a Shortage of Mental-Health Professionals in the U.S.," New York Magazine, Posted October 27, 2015, http://nymag.com/scienceofus/2015/10/theres-a-shortage-of-therapists-in-the-us.html.

like wilderness therapy, weekly psychotherapy for months or years if necessary, and assistance with real life issues like building supportive relationships and finding and keeping employment and housing?

It takes time, whether through in-patient or out-patient care, to explore and ultimately understand the root cause of a patient's mental health obstacles. Perhaps there's a medical issue contributing to the depression such as a thyroid or other hormone imbalance. Maybe a substance dependency hasn't been addressed, or there's trauma and grief from the past. Nutrition plays a huge role in behavioral health, so diet must be on the front lines of discussion and action. Neuroscientists, psychiatrists, and psychologists are slowly opening up to the idea that our gut health is related to our mental health. The gut is sometimes referred to as our "second brain" since the two are connected by an extensive network of neurons. Through this network, chemicals and hormones constantly provide feedback about how hungry we are, if we're stressed, or if we've ingested an unwanted microbe. The expression "trust your gut" is credible in a variety of ways.

IBS (irritable bowel syndrome) is a modern syndrome that affects both the gut and the brain. It is depression in the gut. A person with IBS is likely to feel better when stress management is included in the wellness plan. Some doctors even prescribe antidepressants to treat IBS. For over 50 years, naturopaths have been saying, "Treat the gut. Treat the gut. Treat the gut," and that includes making sure things are flowing in and out of the body, daily. Poop is a waste product of digestion, and regularly eliminating waste promotes a clean and clear intestinal tract and fosters a clean and clear emotional tract. Hopefully, the psychiatrist of the future will either engage in a conversation around diet and gut health or have another professional in the office do so. This seems imperative because a healthy gut often equals a healthy state of mind.

A HEALTHY GUT OFTEN EQUALS A HEALTHY STATE OF MIND.

Treating depression and anxiety is not an easy task for the patient or the physician, nor is it an easy task for any individual to coexist with these states of mind. Mental health conditions rarely disappear for good, but depression and anxiety can be managed properly and effectively by creating a healthy gut, supplementing judiciously, reducing stress, exercising, and when necessary, medicating. I talk to my patients about "learning to dance with their mental health." At times it's a waltz or a line dance and at other times a mosh pit. It's important to gain the insight and skills to "dance" and "move" with emotions so they don't overtake your life. Of course, there are many shades of mental health, and it's essential to have the assistance of well-trained professionals, as well as the support of friends and family.

If you are experiencing anxiety, depression, or panic attacks, I encourage you to share what you are dealing with and not hide it. Let your community know what you are experiencing. When patients begin sharing with their close friends the isolation of their depression, their ability to navigate ups and downs increases. Pregnant women and new moms are especially vulnerable to depression and anxiety. If you know of one in your community, please reach out to her. Let her know you are there to offer emotional support and an hour or two of babysitting, so she can enjoy a nap or a restorative walk in nature.

The more we speak our truth, not just to family and friends, but also to healthcare professionals, the sooner we will become a healthier nation mentally and physically. If you feel anxious or depressed, if you are stressed or panicked, demand that your doctor listen to you and provide options before these conditions lead to poor digestion, thyroid disease, ulcers, substance abuse, or unwarranted medication. Ultimately, healthcare professionals should be creating wellness plans for healthy people who want to remain healthy, not helping people manage diseases.

———————

CHAPTER 13 HEALTH RESOLUTION

What disease(s) run in your family? If you don't know, learn the health histories of your parents, grandparents, great grandparents, and siblings. If you're adopted, see if you can find health-related information on your biological parents. Information is preventative medicine. If you know your family is predisposed to heart disease, diabetes, dementia, addiction, or depression, you can take preventative action. Don't let this information scare you; let it prepare and guide you. Let it be the impetus you may need to make favorable changes in your environment, the food you eat, the way you deal with stress, and the people with whom you keep company. Visit your licensed healthcare professional and ask for information and the creation of a wellness plan complete with preventative measures.

INFORMATION IS PREVENTATIVE MEDICINE.

I have learned the following about my family's health history and have shared it with my trusted healthcare professional:

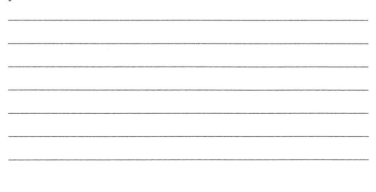

CHAPTER 14

The Health Revolution Solution

As a naturopathic doctor, I hear patients expressing a multitude of frustrations regarding current healthcare options. All too often, they're given only limited time with their doctors. Too many health-related questions are left unanswered, and no comprehensive health plan or goals are set. People don't want to wait until they have a disease and then figure out how to live with it. They want to set up a healthful lifestyle proactively and live fully without having chronic illness enter into the picture.

Over the past twelve years, I have had the opportunity to assist thousands of patients and their families to better understand why they're exhausted, depressed, gaining weight, lacking motivation, anxious, craving junk food, and dealing with too many adverse symptoms. People are tired of just "surviving" and want to know how they can positively affect their health and live better lives daily—without an ever-growing list of medication. People want aha moments regarding the state of their health. If we can heal ourselves gently and effectively, we can heal the Earth, and in turn, the Earth will nurture us. It all comes back to *the Vis*.

I have put forth in this book eight guidelines that I know will help you find and maintain optimum health: 1) Drink lots of water, and 2) eat real food. 3) Ideally, do this with the people, the community, you love. 4) Move around in a way that is joyful, not laborious. 5) If you feel something is not right in your body, investigate. Schedule appropriate lab work to be done. 6) Determine if your hormones are balanced. 7) Check with your trusted, licensed healthcare professional to see if supplementation is necessary. 8) Finally, and most significantly, don't forget to get para. Schedule down time, if you must. Chill. Enjoy nature. Relax. Breathe. Ponder where you fit in the expanse of it all. Experience and revel in your aha moments.

Despite different religious or spiritual beliefs, I think we can all agree that each of us has a concrete number of years to exist on earth in this lifetime. I also think it would be fair to say that we all hope to spend those years in fulfilling ways. We want to be happy as often as we can and enjoy time with others. And, we want to inhabit animated, dynamic bodies on a thriving planet—but to do so, each of us has to take that first step.

A former teacher of mine, Dr. Bill Mitchell, ND, said, "Your future health begins now." For each of us, there are decisions to make nearly every single moment. "Do I buy that double cappuccino my mind says I need to make it through the second half of the day, or do I drink a big glass of water with fresh squeezed lemon juice?" "Do I watch three hours of TV in the evening, or do I share a meal with a neighbor followed by a neighborhood stroll?" "Do I accept taking medications for life, or do I search for and demand alternatives?" "Do I go to the bathroom when my body signals it's time to go, or do I hold it because I'm too busy?" Nearly every choice we make has some impact on our physical, emotional, and spiritual health. We can be passive and allow the current disease-based model to persist in healthcare, or we can be vocal and active and work to change the way we do health in America. We can be part of The Health Revolution. We can transform our healthcare system into one that is focused on prevention and thereby become a healthy nation instead of a sick one.

NEARLY EVERY CHOICE WE MAKE HAS SOME IMPACT ON OUR PHYSICAL, EMOTIONAL, AND SPIRITUAL HEALTH.

I urge you to become a vibrant participant in The Health Revolution. Become active in your community, socially and politically. Request reimbursement for integrative healthcare from you insurance provider. Work with a doctor who listens to *you* and develops a comprehensive wellness plan. Conduct business with local organic farmers. Let all the aha moments you have during this health-seeking venture inspire your divine purpose.

Made in the USA
Las Vegas, NV
09 January 2022